MW01236181

HOW TO ELIMINATE
THE Yo Yo EFFECT
IN WEIGHT LOSS

Dori Luneski, R.N., N.D.

authorHOUSE®

AuthorHouse™
1663 Liberty Drive
Bloomington, IN 47403
www.authorhouse.com
Phone: 1-800-839-8640

Published by AuthorHouse 5/4/2012

ISBN: 978-1-4685-4611-8 (sc)
ISBN: 978-1-4685-4610-1 (e)

DISCLAIMER

HOW TO ELIMINATE THE YO YO EFFECT IN WEIGHT LOSS is not intended to treat disease, in any way interfere with diagnostic procedures or treatment by any medical practitioner, or be construed as medical advice. This book may seem controversial to some; it is not intended to satisfy modern science. The opinions herein are strictly those of the author. The "first do no harm" recommendations in this book are meant to be guidelines to assist the body to work at optimal performance, or heal itself if possible. Even in the face of serious illness, the principles of wellness should not be ignored. The author urges anyone having a health concern to see a licensed practitioner for evaluation. The application of any concepts in this book without the consent of a licensed practitioner is not encouraged; however, it is your constitutional right to decide how you wish to treat your body. The author and the publisher assume no liability for the implementation of any material presented.

ACKNOWLEDGMENTS

To …

Eddie Archuleta, my husband, who supports me in everything I do, and is my best friend. He is always helpful when I need a second opinion on any subject.

To …

Patrice Luneski, who inspired me to read many weight loss books that made it obvious another weight loss book needed to be written. This book deals with specific issues not covered in other weight loss books.

To …

Dan Luneski, who is the best part of a support team any writer could have, whether an idea or a computer problem.

FOREWORD

By Marianne Rothschild M.D.

Finally, thanks to this wonderful book by Dr. Dori Luneski, we finally have a serious and thorough delineation of the holistic approach to weight loss.

Dr. Dori gives us guidelines that include all four pillars of wellness as they relate to weight loss. Weight loss will never result in permanent change if we fail to address the physical, mental, emotional and spiritual aspects of a human being's life. And healthy weight is the result of healthy being.

So many weight loss programs fail to address the deeper issues involved in living a life in balance. As Dr. Luneski so clearly explains, the real issue is not LOSING WEIGHT but achieving and sustaining a healthy way of living.

We Americans have become accustomed to the "quick fix". We look for immediate gratification and focus our plans on short term solutions. This approach has not worked in the past and shows no hope for working in the future. How long are we going to continue to do the same thing and expect a different result? The definition for that is stupidity or perhaps even insanity.

In the face of weight loss insanity, Dr. Luneski offers us a sane and a refreshingly clear step by step format for achieving and maintaining wellness. Who better to teach us then Dr. Dori? I personally know many people she has helped recover from devastating illnesses or a lifetime of disability through her wise holistic guidance. This book provides an opportunity for many to benefit from her years of experience and wisdom.

There are no short cuts to weight loss just as there are no short cuts to health. Achieving a healthy weight is the result of a body, mind and spirit in harmony and there are no short cuts. Thank you Dr. Dori!

INTRODUCTION

You are reading this page because you want to lose weight. It could be five pounds, ten pounds, fifty pounds or more. *This is probably not your first attempt at losing weight.* You may have had some success in the past with a weight loss plan. You may be thrilled to finally fit into that little polka dot bikini . . . but you may still be stuffy from allergies . . . or your joints may hurt . . . or you gained the weight back after you went off the diet plan. You may have diligently followed every recommendation in a number of weight loss books. You may own most weight loss books looking for that magic plan that works for you. You may have tried every expert's opinion as to why their book is the last weight loss book you will ever need to read. *And yet, here you are reading this book.*

By now you may be tired of the confusion of *high* this and *low* that in one book and the opposite in another book. You've exercised faithfully, eaten healthier food than you've ever eaten, and grown tired of calorie counting and that intimidating measuring cup. Most of all you may be tired of the whole subject of weight loss that seems to dominate your life. Considering all your focus on weight loss, you may be disappointed that losing weight does not always mean you are free of nagging symptoms of poor health. You may be so excited you lost some weight that you do not care as much about the headaches, chronic pain, hyperactivity or fatigue, or any one of a dozen other symptoms people *live with and tolerate every day.*

I will not insult your intelligence by saying that this is the last weight loss book you will ever have to read. You've heard that before

... too many times. What I want to do is to activate your intellectual curiosity to look at elements of weight loss that are generally not discussed in traditional approaches of losing the pounds and inches. Yes, I will discuss water and exercise. Yes, I will discuss healthy eating choices. Yes, I will discuss basic rules of dieting you probably already know . . . but what you may not know is in this book, and that could be the difference between short term or long term success **OF NOT JUST WEIGHT LOSS BUT A SENSE OF WELL BEING!**

You are on a journey of filling in valuable information that makes the usual weight loss plan fit *your biochemical individuality.* Tomatoes and other nightshade foods discussed in this book are not good for everyone if you have joint pains. Almonds and other salicylate foods discussed in this book are not good for everyone if you are *chemically* sensitive to those foods. Dairy discussed in this book is not good for everyone if you do not have strong adrenals that deal with stress and allergic reactions. Red meat and other acid forming foods discussed in this book are not good for everyone if your pH (body chemistry) is too acidic. Mango and other tropical fruits discussed in this book are not good for everyone if you do not process fructose well. **Too many books in print do not deal with YOUR individual personal state of wellness or disease in recommending diet plans and recipes.** *This book is different!!!* You will be taught all the health tips that *make YOUR choices work for YOU AS AN INDIVIDUAL . . . not just now, but for your lifetime.*

You've heard the saying, "You get what you pay for." Quality does count, and the definition of quality is excellence. You can only have excellence in your effort to lose weight if you have all the facts about how EVERY CHOICE you make affects **YOUR BODY.** Millions of people may read a weight loss book that is hot on the market. However, not everybody is the same, so individualizing your weight loss plan is critical. Get ready for an exciting journey of **more** than weight loss. Get ready for a slimmer body that is also capable of staying healthy.

GET READY TO INDIVIDUALIZE YOUR WEIGHT LOSS PLAN!!!

We are in this journey together … **SO TURN THE PAGE AND CHANGE YOUR LIFE!!!**

Dori Luneski, RN, Naturopathic Practitioner

Contents

WATER

Starting your weight loss plan means thinking about a critical element of health protection … a healthy drinking water source. That source should be easily available in your home. You should not have to run to the grocery store if you are out of safe water. *That makes it likely you will either substitute unsafe water or drink less than you should to stretch what water you have available.* You can have **filtered spring** water (not filtered tap water) delivered to your home. Or consider buying a reverse osmosis water filtration unit for your home. I prefer reverse osmosis over other filtering units because it back washes the filters with each use. This back washing makes the filtration reliable longer than filters that collect residue from the first use until replaced. Most commercial water filtering units that fit on your faucet may only take out chlorine and some heavy metals. The water tastes better, but commercial water filtration systems will not remove fluoride, parasites, some heavy metals, chemicals and drugs in city water. Distilled water has no molecular energy, is very acidic and can flush out good nutrients. ALL FILTERED WATER LOSES ELECTROLYTES … SO MAKE SURE YOU ADD ELECTROLYTE DROPS TO ANY FILTERED WATER. Check your health food store for electrolyte drops that put the energy back into filtered water.

One source of healthy water that contains all the electrolytes is **100% Pure Coconut Water (without any added ingredients)**. This water comes from the young green coconuts and is more hydrating and alkalizing than even energized filtered water. Coconut Water is the same composition as human blood plasma and was used during the 2nd World War for blood plasma. It is most economical if you purchase by the case with the case discount from your health food store, Amazon.com, or Vitacost.com. Do not consume in excess as too many electrolytes can be hard on the kidneys to eliminate from the body. Drinking ½ -1 cup a day in place of that amount of energized filtered water is a recommended amount to add quality hydration and alkalinity to your program. **Do not add extra electrolyte drops to coconut water.** You may not need coconut water if your urine and saliva pH is above 6.6. If your pH is below 6.6 on urine and saliva, you can *start* using coconut water … once your pH reaches 6.6 and above on both urine and saliva, you can *stop* using coconut water.

We are composed of 70 % water, 85% in the brain cells. Water volume in your spinal discs supports 75% of the weight in your upper body. Cartilage in joints and discs are 50% water. *The digestive system is ineffective without correct water.* Symptoms or pain anywhere in the body can be a sign of local cellular thirst. *Some people have cellular dehydration because they flush everything out from over hydration. Too much of a good thing does not make it better.* **THE FUNCTIONING OF YOUR WHOLE BODY ON A DAILY BASIS DEPENDS ON CORRECT HYDRATION OF CELLS BASED ON 1 OUNCE FOR EVERY 2 POUNDS OF BODY WEIGHT… UNLESS GENETICALLY YOU ARE A HYDRIPHERIC TYPE WHO HOLDS TOO MUCH WATER OUTSIDE THE CELLS. IF YOU ARE OVERWEIGHT, SWELL EASILY IN YOUR ARMS AND LEGS IF YOU DRINK TOO MUCH WATER, AND HAVE OVERWEIGHT RELATIVES YOU SHOULD LIMIT YOUR WATER TO 8-9 GLASSES DAILY.** If you are concerned about being a hydripheric type you can go to any library and read more on the subject in "The Chemistry of Man" by Bernard Jensen, or in my book "The Power to Heal."

THE SENSATION OF THIRST AND HUNGER ARE GENERATED SIMULTANEOUSLY IN THE BRAIN. We eat food even when the body is really asking for water. To lose weight you need to understand that the brain uses two mechanisms for its

energy requirements. **The first is from the breakdown of food and the manufacturing of sugar in the liver if there is not enough sugar in your circulation. The second mechanism is from the water supply and conversion of hydroelectric energy.** The brain is *overactive* and *dehydrated* in times of stress. *Because modern America produces stress we did not have even 50 years ago, the overactive brain in modern times requires daily maintenance. If the body does not supply the sugar needs due to an unhealthy liver, you will give into eating more often, and in larger quantities.* We tend to gain weight in an unending effort to supply the brain with energy. However, not all food energy reaches the brain. *If exercise does not burn up overindulged sugar, it is stored in the muscles as fat.* **When you use water as the source of brain energy instead of sugar, you will not have muscle storage of excess sugar. Excess water is passed out in your urine that does not create the problem associated with excess sugar.**

Water deserves top billing where health is concerned … it must be a major consideration in any weight loss program. Dehydration is the **number one stressor** of the human body or of any living matter … try not watering your plants and see what happens. **Water controls free movement of molecules, so exchange of nutrients and elimination of toxins can occur that is critical in your weight loss program.** *We mistakenly assume that all fluid is equivalent to water. This assumption could be the basis of many chronic health problems … including weight gain.* Caffeine products have addictive properties, are diuretics and are dehydrating agents. Because you think you have consumed enough water after a soda or coffee, when you get those hunger signs you assume you need to eat … and that may be more food than your body needs. WHAT YOUR BODY NEEDED WAS WATER! *So… dehydration caused by caffeine containing drinks can cause gradual weight gain from overeating* **as a direct result of your body being confused with the thirst and hunger sensations of the brain.**

An important reflex that occurs in the brain is a reaction to sweet taste. If the sweet taste in **artificially** sweetened products is not followed by **natural** nutrient availability of healthy sweets, *the urge to eat will be the outcome.* **The more sweet taste without the calories to stimulate the**

taste buds, the more urge to eat … and eat … and eat. *Drinking diet soda has become a fad in this country obsessed with overweight concerns. 'Diet' soda sounds better, but you cannot fool Mother Nature and get away with it!!!* **One of the biggest mistakes you can make in your quest for weight loss is not to know the difference between fluids and healthy fluids or water!!!**

Our industrial society has severely compromised our water with high levels of inorganic minerals, toxins, heavy metals, chemicals and drugs. Too often we do not understand that the lack of the most important element in the human body … healthy water … can clog any system or organ and generate pain and illness. **Increased water intake gives you energy.** The daily walking we talk about later stimulates the production of enzymes that cleans your circulatory system. **A HEALTHY CIRCULATORY SYSTEM IS A MAJOR FIRST STEP IN WEIGHT MANAGEMENT!**

MAKE THE WATER YOU DRINK THE BEST IT CAN BE! Lately, even some hard plastic containers are controversial, so to be safe, carry water in stainless steel or glass … or plastic bottles that are BPA free and do not have a plain #7 on the bottom. *Carry filtered and energized drinking water with you wherever you go…shopping, restaurant or to work.*

THIS IS YOUR LIFE… IT IS NOT A REHEARSAL! With your health education developing daily as you read this book, you will learn how to take care of your body … *so when you get where you are going, not just your slimmer body, but your SLIMMER HEALTHY BODY will be there with you. REMEMBER, IF YOU LOSE WEIGHT AND ARE NOT HEALTHY, YOU WILL PROBABLY GAIN IT BACK. IF YOU ARE BASICALLY HEALTHY, YOU SHOULD LOSE WEIGHT NATURALLY WITHOUT ONE DIET PLAN AFTER ANOTHER, COMPLICATED INSTRUCTIONS OR HIGH THIS AND LOW THAT! Read on … your lifetime weight loss health plan just keeps getting better!!!*

WEIGHT LOSS TIP #2

BODY PH BALANCE

The Chinese knew about pH 5,000 years ago and called it yin-yang, or the balance of the life force. **IT IS ALL ABOUT BALANCE!!!** When imbalance occurs, we start building any symptom in the human body that can *range from* poor digestion, low energy, aches and pains, poor concentration and the dreaded weight gain. Fat cells carry acids away from vital organs in an attempt to protect them … and that is one reason why your body does not want to lose the fat. *This book is not just about a slimmer body, but it is also about the biggest bonus of all … which is regaining your health.* While diet may be the key to weight loss, *it has to be a diet that balances your body chemistry.* **MORE IMPORTANT THAN COUNTING CALORIES AND FAT GRAMS IN YOUR EFFORT TO LOSE WEIGHT, IS TESTING YOUR URINE AND SALIVA PH TO DETERMINE BODY CHEMISTRY BALANCE!!!**

The nature of the human body is governed by bio-electrical energy that ranges from acidity to alkalinity. For proper body functions an acid-alkaline balance must be maintained. ***Do not focus on weight loss without understanding if your body is capable of the balance needed to support and maintain your goal, now and in the future.*** In low resistance to chronic illness that includes weight fluctuations, your system may be too alkaline or too acidic. In poor stress management plus the typical American diet and lifestyle, acidity dominates. If you want more technical information about pH you can get books to explain the chemistry behind pH (pronounced like the two letters) that reflects the concentration of positively charged molecules in any solution. ***What you need to know now** is that acids and alkalis are opposites, and their meeting should cancel each other out creating a neutral 7 pH.*

If the urine and saliva pH measurements are not in the best range of 6.6-7.0, it does not matter what illness is present. *Calling the illness weight gain and cutting carbohydrates or implementing other weight loss programs will not successfully keep the weight off if you have not corrected pH imbalance.* **DO NOT FOCUS ON VARIOUS PRINCIPLES OF WEIGHT LOSS AND IGNORE AN IMBALANCED PH!!!** It does not matter how you got to where you are … never forget that a good organic, mostly plant based diet and a positive attitude about your life's situations help turn your body chemistry around. Eating the right kind of food to balance your pH is the most important thing you can do for your wellness effort. *This whole book is designed to help you develop a life changing dietary and wellness plan that you are comfortable enough to stay with for a lifetime … and not just focusing on a short term weight loss plan.*

School children get their school supplies before school starts, and since you are in your own version of the *school of life*, you also need supplies. That means you need pH testing paper. One contact for pH testing paper is 1-718-338-3618 or www.microessentiallab.com. All pH testing paper is the same in that it tests the pH of whatever liquid you are testing. Some pH testing products are more expensive than others because they read other values besides pH, like in diabetic testing supplies. All you need is the least expensive paper that tests the broadest range for easier reading. The pH paper used to test swimming pools or fish tanks is not calibrated fine enough for human data. All pH paper comes with a color chart. The lighter green to yellow color indicates acidity and the darker green indicates alkalinity. You want to be in the medium green with both urine and saliva. *Urine and saliva pH should both be in the medium green range of 6.6–7.0. If both urine and saliva are more than a .5 difference between the two readings your body is too stressed to function correctly. For either urine or saliva testing, 6.4 is starting to be too acidic and over 7.2 is too alkaline.* **Body pH does not**

straighten out overnight, so be patient and follow each **WEIGHT LOSS TIP** outlined in this book for your long term success story.

Without correct pH you may not get the value of expensive supplements or organic food as much as you think you should from the effort you are making. **THE PH OF YOUR URINE AND SALIVA TELLS YOU IF WHAT YOU ARE DOING IS WORKING FOR YOU . . . OR NOT . . . SO PAY ATTENTION TO THIS IMPORTANT AND INFORMATIVE BODY LANGUAGE!** These health tips are not intended to teach you all you need to know about this subject, but they should introduce you to important health information you can choose to learn more about. *There are excellent books that deal with the subject of balancing your body chemistry. To get you started consider the following:*

IF YOUR URINE IS BELOW 6.6 YOU ARE ACIDIC:

- *Make sure you take a **buffered vitamin C supplement** and not ascorbic acid.*

- *Based on individual tolerance to foods **eat more alkaline forming foods** like...*

*All **sprouted** grains*	***Unrefined** oils*
Millet, quinoa, amaranth	***Unrefined** natural sea salt*
All vegetables, fresh beans	*Fruits except cranberry, plum, prunes and blueberries*
Herbal teas	*Cooking herbs and spices*
Almonds	*Brown rice syrup*
Raw apple cider vinegar	*Sweet brown rice vinegar*

- ***No smoking.***

- *Consider **Sun Chlorella** brand of chlorophyll.*

- *Take vegetarian formulas of **digestive enzymes**.*

- *No caffeine except green tea.*

- *Stress increases acidity. If you are not handling stress well, research homeopathic formulas for stress, and take a **natural food based B Complex** such as the one made by MegaFood available in health food stores..*

- ***Increase exercise.***

- *Drink **organic vegetable juice** available in health food stores. If you have joint pains you may not be handling the nightshade foods well and cannot tolerate the tomatoes in vegetable juices. You can make your own blender drink based on tolerated vegetables that will be discussed later in this book.*

IF YOUR URINE IS ABOVE 7.2 YOU ARE TOO ALKALINE:

- *You may be dumping alkaline minerals from **too many alkaline foods or supplements.** Your Vitamin C product should be ascorbic acid.*

- *You may be eating too high acidic diet so the body tries to alkalize the system by pulling calcium from the bones, and **excess calcium is discarded in the urine.** Reduce your intake of acid forming proteins (especially beef and veal, pork, buffalo, deer and lamb) and grains that are not sprouted.*

IF YOUR SALIVA IS BELOW 6.6 YOU ARE TOO ACIDIC:

- *Take dairy free vegetarian based **digestive enzymes** with each meal.*

- *Evaluate **stress management** and reduce stress around mealtime.*

- Drink a glass of **water before you start to eat each meal,** no water with the meal and no water ½ hour after the meal.

- **Eat slower and chew your food well.**

- Take 2 dairy free, vegetarian **probiotic** capsules (good bacteria for the digestive system) every morning at least 30 minutes before breakfast.

- Eat 3 meals a day, **do not skip meals** and do not eat after 8 PM.

- Use a **buffered Vitamin C supplement** instead of ascorbic acid for your Vitamin C supplement.

IF YOUR SALIVA IS ABOVE 7.2 YOU ARE TOO ALKALINE:

- Based on your individual tolerance to certain foods, increase your intake of **acid forming foods** such as:

Eggs	Chicken
Fish/seafood	Ostrich/Emu
Duck	Peanuts
Nuts	Dried beans

- Take **hydrochloric acid with pepsin tablets** with each protein meal and dairy free vegetarian based digestive enzymes with each meal.

- Improve **elimination** to have a good bowel movement daily before noon.

- **Drink a glass of water before eating,** no water with the meal and no water ½ hour after the meal.

- Take **ascorbic acid for your Vitamin C product.**

Dori Luneski, R.N., N.D.

Weight loss should be a side benefit, because what you really want to achieve is a healthier body. CONGRATULATIONS … YOU ARE THE MIRACLE OF THE MOMENT BUILDING A HEALTHIER BODY THAT MAKES YOUR WEIGHT LOSS PROGRAM SUCCESSFUL NOW … AND KEEPS BEING A SUCCESS STORY IN THE FUTURE!

A HEALTHY BODY WILL MAINTAIN ITS OWN IDEAL WEIGHT NATURALLY!!!

WHEN YOU ALKALIZE… YOU ENERGIZE!!!

The reason disease is skyrocketing in spite of all our medical breakthroughs is simple … most people suffer from ACID OVERLOAD. *The typical American diet is acid-forming … meats, eggs, refined bread, milk and cheese, coffee, chocolate, sugar, rice, cereal, cookies, crackers, cakes, pies, candy, sugary drinks, processed foods etc., etc., etc.* All that food we crave and love from the coffee and donut for breakfast to the pizza for dinner, added to over the counter and prescription drugs produces over-acidification of body fluids and tissues. *Acidity is linked in some way to **EVERY KNOWN DISEASE** including the ever popular fibromyalgia, chronic fatigue, digestive and elimination problems . . . and weight gain.*

America is a run-a-way train when it comes to health and wellness. **ONLY YOU CAN DECIDE ENOUGH IS ENOUGH. ONLY YOU CAN SAY YOU ARE TIRED OF BEING SICK AND TIRED, AND REALLY TIRED OF THE MERRY-GO-ROUND OF WEIGHT LOSS SUGGESTIONS. ONLY YOU CAN TAKE CHARGE OF YOUR LIFE AND CHOOSE TO MAKE RESPONSIBLE CHOICES. ONLY YOU CAN CHOOSE NOT TO PUT MONEY IN THE POCKETS OF PROFESSIONALS WHO DO NOT GIVE YOU ENOUGH VALUABLE AND CORRECT INFORMATION TO STAY WELL.**

Read any book on health and wellness and you will read about the value of *green food* that is **more** than just green vegetables. **Organic green food and super food supplements *along with* organic vegetables helps you break the acid overload cycle.** These modern miracle foods that carry off acids and flush them through your kidneys may be your 1st line of defense against fatigue, illness, disease . . . and weight gain. Green is the color of healthy plants that provide you with new cellular growth and healing. **Healthy green food keeps giving seriously high nutrient levels squeezed into a ridiculously small space.** *It is called more bang for your buck!!!* If financial stress is messing up your day, help your body cope with stress by considering organic food and supplements over commercial formulas you may not be absorbing.

The best supplements are not made chemically in a laboratory. The body will always accept natural food better than synthetic fractions of nutrients in a commercial supplement formulated in a chemist's lab. **ALL SUPER-FOOD PRODUCTS PROVIDE HIGHLY ABSORBABLE NUTRIENTS THAT SUPPORTS THE BODY TO WORK AT OPTIMUM PERFORMANCE AND HEAL ITSELF IF POSSIBLE.** When shopping for supplements look for words like vegetarian, organic, natural food or whole food. *Learn to shop smart when selecting your supplement program.*

Being overweight is at least partly due to insufficient enzymes to correctly transform and utilize food. Superior natural enzyme activity comes from natural whole foods. Healthy cells love oxygen, and any chlorophyll rich food oxygenates the blood. Always remember to keep it simple!!! **Here are some *super food* facts to support your effort for a slimmer, healthier body:**

1. **Spirulina** is an algae that contains 70 percent protein and all the essential amino acids. Spirulina is the highest known vegetable source of B12, and is an excellent choice for a totally natural super food supplement. It is so complete in all basic nutrients you could survive with just Spirulina and water. Look for organic Spirulina for consistent nutritional content. You can take Spirulina as capsules with water … or

just toss the vegetable capsules or bulk Spirulina powder into a blender drink to provide inexpensive natural nutrition.

2. **Barley and Wheat Grass** may be the fast food of the future. Millions of people are now drinking grass for their health … not the kind in your yard. Concentrated grass juice is dehydrated to a powder at low temperatures allowing the enzymes to remain alive. All the nutrients, chlorophyll, enzymes, vitamins and minerals are balanced by nature and absorbed directly through cell membranes in the digestive system. These grass products have been promoted for decades for purifying the blood and detoxifying the liver. *But not every good suggestion is tolerated by every person.* If you have any bloating, gas, irritable bowel, colitis or any other bowel disorder you may NOT want to start with these *gluten grains* until your intestinal symptoms improve. In all people with chronic intestinal symptoms grains may be a problem, but *organic sprouted grains* may be more tolerated.

3. The best brand for superior absorption of chlorella is **Sun Chlorella**, a *tiny dark green pill with the highest chlorophyll level of the green foods and screams out health just looking at it!!!* Sun Chlorella is a single celled chlorophyll algae that is grown under controlled surroundings in large pools of pure mineral water producing a beneficial health building nutrient and cellular cleanser. Sun Chlorella has a patented process of breaking down the cell wall for maximum digestion and absorption. It is highly recommended to alkalize an acidic pH. This easy to digest form of chlorella also acts like an *adaptogen* that helps your body become more resistant to environmental and health stresses.

4. **Bee Pollen** contains certain enzymes which are essential catalysts to aid in digestion. Bee Pollen is capable of its own digestion and aids digestion of other foods. It contains up to 30 percent protein, plus essential sugars, vitamins and

minerals in a natural perfect food form. As one of the richest foods in nature, Bee Pollen contains every basic ingredient needed to sustain life ... so do not forget to consider it as part of your natural supplement program. Do not take Bee Pollen is you have had a severe reaction to bee stings.

5. **Brewer's Yeast** is more than a treasure house of nutrients. It is truly nature's wonder-food! It is one of the best natural sources of the entire B complex needed for digestion and stress management. It is a superb source of concentrated complete protein, rich in essential fatty acids and trace minerals. It is the best nutritional source of Chromium in an organic compound known as GTF (glucose Tolerance Factor). GTF is essential for the production of functionally effective insulin. Brewer's Yeast varies greatly based on how it is grown. Lewis Laboratories Premium Brewer's Yeast is grown on Sugar Beets, and does not have the same negative taste of yeast grown on hops or grain. Since Lewis Laboratory Brewer's Yeast is not an active yeast food it does not produce the same concerns for people with Candida yeast symptoms. This better tasting easy to digest super food can be added to any liquid for additional nutrients.

6. **Coconut Secret** products do not taste like coconut because they come from the sap of the tree and not the coconut. This line of products has a very low glycemic index of 35, is diabetic friendly, an abundant source of minerals, 17 amino acids, vitamin C, broad-spectrum B vitamins, and has a nearly neutral pH. Use the **Coconut Aminos** in place of soy sauce for favoring ... the **Coconut vinegar** is a fabulous substitution of grain or apple based vinegar if you have problems with those foods ... the granulated **Coconut Crystals** can substitute for the same amount of brown or white sugar ... and the liquid **Coconut Nectar** can replace maple syrup or other high glycemic sugars in baking or other sweet needs. These products make calorie reducing easy!!! You do not have to give up your favorite recipes if

you substitute these products for high glycemic or poorly tolerated foods.

Remember, I'm **super** energetic at age 78 … **I LOVE SUPER FOODS AND TRUST MY HEALTH TO NATURE!!!**

WEIGHT LOSS TIP # 4

EXERCISE

You are starting one of the most important segments of your life journey ... *control over who you are on all levels of spiritual, mental, emotional and physical.* ***YOU ARE AN INDIVIDUAL WITH YOUR OWN PERSONAL ISSUES***. *Because there are no two people exactly alike, you will need personal guidance to assist you in making **your** journey successful.* If I told you to eat a banana split each day to lose weight you would love my book. As a society we want choices to be easy and fun. **HEALTHY CHOICES CAN BE EASY ... AND FUN!!!**

School age children love exercise without realizing their joy and deep breathing are healthy. Too often playful children turn into serious, goal-oriented adults. Losing that youthful enthusiasm for life makes it more difficult as an adult to establish exercise habits just for pleasure. Many adults exercise for social, business or undesirable health issues. Hopefully, by the time you finish this book you will exercise not only for the health benefits, but also because ***exercise produces endorphins that just plain make you feel better.***

John Kennedy said, "Ask not what your country can do for you. Ask what you can do for your country." So stop asking what your body can do for you, and start thinking about what nice things you can do for your body. **IT IS NOT IMPORTANT WHAT YOU PLAY ... IT IS JUST IMPORTANT THAT YOU PLAY!!!** *Play may be the most vital thing you do.* Weight loss books recommend exercise for weight control. But exercise is also stressed for poor circulation, constipation and a list of other symptoms nobody wants. *THIS CAN HARDLY BE*

CONSIDERED FUN. **FITNESS SHOULD BE A LOT MORE THAN PREVENTING DISEASE OR LOSING WEIGHT. FITNESS SHOULD BE DOING SOMETHING NICE FOR YOUR BODY. NEVER FORGET THAT THE HUMAN BODY IS TRULY A MIRACLE.** When you open your eyes each morning think about the miracle of being alive. **THIS IS YOUR DAY! WHAT ARE YOU GOING TO DO WITH IT?**

THIS MAY BE THE MOST IMPORTANT WEIGHT LOSS PARAGRAPH YOU WILL EVER READ IN ANY WEIGHT LOSS BOOK!!! Your decision to exercise or make healthy choices is based on more than your physical condition. It is based on your **TOTAL WELLNESS ON ALL LEVELS OF MENTAL, EMOTIONAL AND PHYSICAL.** You may not have any physical limitations, but if you have mental (thinking) or emotional (feeling) issues *YOU JUST DO NOT CARE TO EXERCISE OR MAKE OTHER GOOD CHOICES.* Negative emotions or negative thinking can interfere with your *enthusiasm* even if you are free of physical symptoms. This loss of *enthusiasm* can make you less motivated regardless of the encouragement to exercise or eat differently in your latest weight loss book. Acute symptoms are usually on the physical level, but most other times symptoms are mental and emotional as well as physical. **Learn how all these levels influence your life and it will help you understand why you make good choices ... or bad choices ... why some days you are proud of what you do and your self-esteem is high ... and other days you know you could have done better and your self-esteem is low.**

"Self-esteem isn't everything. It is just that there is nothing without it."

-Gloria Swanson

The best place to start is to look at exercise as a way of adding *pleasure* to your day. When exercise produces those feel good endorphins, you will look at the stressors of the day with a more *positive attitude.* The success of your exercise program does not depend on how many exercise books, tapes or weight loss books you read . . . but success does depend on your **FRAME OF MIND!** Make a *commitment* to your future, and experience a private satisfaction that you are doing something for **YOU**. If **YOU** cannot give **YOU** part of each day, look at the value you place on yourself. *YOUR WEIGHT GAIN MAY NOT BE YOUR PROBLEM!!! YOUR PROBLEM MAY BE THE CHOICES YOU MAKE BASED ON THE VALUE YOU PLACE ON YOURSELF … AND THAT SAYS IT ALL!!!*

Today the weight loss tip is exercise that moves the *lymphatic system … your "Doctor" within that cleans up toxic wastes*. It is your lymphatic system that cleans the blood. That means 30 minutes **MINIMUM 6-7 days a week of nonstop walking type exercise**. You might get away with 6 days a week … but you will not get enough health benefits from 5 or less days a week. Consider any choice that impacts the bottom of the feet like walking, trampoline, treadmill, etc. It is NOT recommended that you jog or run at this stage. You may not be fully hydrated with enough water … and that can take one to two months of drinking correctly. Dehydration can be hard on the joints that are all cushioned with water. *ABOUT 30 MINUTES OF WALKING TYPE EXERCISE 6-7 DAYS A WEEK THE REST OF YOUR LIFE IS A MUST IF YOU WANT TO ENJOY FEEL GOOD ENERGY, SURVIVE LIVING IN MODERN AMERICA AND MAINTAIN WEIGHT CONTROL!* During part of the walk, give thanks for all the special people and benefits in your life. **Use this private time to focus on your blessings that increases energy … and not what is missing that depletes energy.**

"The dog ate my homework" is nothing compared to the excuses I've heard for not having time to do this important health recommendation. My personal plan for **total compliance** starts when I get up, go to the bathroom, drink a glass of water, take my probiotic good bacteria on an empty stomach and do about 10 minutes of my favorite stretches. I stretch both arms out and **inhale in as much air as possible**… then bring arms around like a hug under the breast area. Firmly pressing the lower lungs I lean forward and push **ALL** the air out. After 5 deep cleansing breaths I start fast walking for 30 minutes through the rooms on the 1st floor of my home. For added muscle tension I walk with three pound weights in each hand. Always remember to thank God with a big smile for the gift of life this day, for the sunny day or rain that is the

miracle of life. If you cannot walk 30 minutes, at least do 10 minutes and increase as tolerated until you can handle 30 minutes. **This daily repetition of stretching, deep breathing and walking helps develop your lifetime habit**. Walking one time a day is necessary for good health, but walking longer than 30 minutes or more than one time a day is helpful in weight loss.

EXERCISE EQUIPMENT TO CONSIDER:

- If you cannot walk, consider a rocking chair allowing your bare feet to impact the hard floor as you rock. This only works well with the old fashion rocker, not the glider chair.

- You may find you can tolerate Pilates or other similar equipment that allows you to exercise lying flat. For some people this may be better than putting your whole body weight pressure on hips, knees or ankles. If you cannot locate this kind of equipment check with QVC, 1-800-354-1515.

- Products like the slant board that can stretch out your muscles, or a balance ball from www.gaiam.com or 1-800-869-3446 can move the lymph. The Healthy Circulation Machine, also from Gaiam catalog rocks the whole body to improve the circulation and the lymphatic system. Check their catalog for many health oriented products. **BEGIN THE DAY WITH ENERGY THAT WILL BENEFIT YOU ALL DAY!**

- A treadmill has become a national favorite for good reason. It allows you to have an excellent indoor walking machine you can use every day, even in bad weather.

- Not everyone has room for big pieces of equipment. Look for a favorite exercise or dance tape you can use in your home for those days you do not want to walk outside, or go to the gym. Dancing to a music tape is a great way to feel good about your body as it wiggles here and there. We all feel better when we 'let go' and loosen up. Check QVC for different exercise or dance exercise tapes.

— Trampolines are great for some people. Women with large breasts may feel uncomfortable jumping. People who have a balance problem should not use a trampoline without a support bar. People who are heavy should only invest in more expensive trampolines that are stronger, as the springs in the small inexpensive version may not hold up for long. Stronger trampolines are also larger, so space is important to consider. You only have to jump one inch to accomplish lymphatic exercise so jumping high is not necessary. Also, always stay in the middle of the trampoline and do not get too foot fancy. I tried to do some fancy dancing on a small trampoline once but I came down on the rim and lost my balance. I hit my head as I fell and never forgot that acting silly on the trampoline can cause accidents.

You will find the time to exercise if that is your choice!!! One lawyer solved his time problem by setting a timer and marching in his office while reading his legal papers. Another lady never had a break once she got to her office. She solved her problem by parking further away, so it took her 30 minutes to get to her office door. Another lady never had a spare minute once her children got up, so she waited until after breakfast, and the youngest children were amused watching her exercise to music with the older ones. *Trying means nothing … when it comes to exercise, you either do or you don't. You get no physical health credit for critically needed energy with only wishful thinking! Figure out what fits your lifestyle and MAKE IT HAPPEN DAILY!* **Smile and have an energetic day … and make someone looking at you also feel better.**

Exercise is an activity that *enriches* the life of a person who has mental, emotional and physical energy enough to be enthusiastic about life. The decision to exercise is based on the decision to *enjoy life to the fullest*. The decision to *begin* exercise *implies* a degree of

health in POSITIVE THINKING, NUTRITION, DIGESTION AND ELIMINATION. The decision to *continue* exercise is a *definite* degree of health in POSITIVE THINKING, NUTRITION, DIGESTION AND ELIMINATION.

"THE FIRST WEALTH IS HEALTH"

...Ralph Waldo Emerson

THIS IS YOUR LIFE ... IT IS NOT A REHEARSAL!

WEIGHT LOSS TIP # 5

SLEEP

You are learning some **basic "laws" of wellness** about water, pH of body chemistry and exercise … now it is time to go to sleep. ***People who are exhausted from lack of sleep are much more likely to make poor decisions in general, and that can sabotage a weight loss program.*** The circadian rhythm for healing occurs between 8 PM and 4 AM when people in past generations used to sleep. You can only heal and regenerate during deep REM (Rapid Eye Movement) sleep. Electricity and technology of modern times discourage most people from getting enough REM sleep to slow the aging process. Going to bed by 10 PM is best, 11 PM is fair. **You should get a minimum of 4 ½ hours of sleep before 4 AM.** *Weight gain is one symptom of general poor health … and unhealthy people do not get enough deep healing sleep.*

In Traditional Chinese Medicine (TCM), any sleep disturbance is seen as a disorder of your spirit. Mind (thinking), body, and spirit (emotional) all need to be evaluated. Sleep comes naturally when you feel grounded in your purpose (not fearful or anxious), and your body is functioning at a high level of performance. **If you wonder what all that means, you should not wonder after reading this book!**

So what do you do if you can't *zzzzzzzzzzzzzzzzzzzzzzz*? Most people do not go to bed when it gets dark or get up with the chickens anymore. *If you have trouble getting to sleep or staying asleep, consider these highly recommended tips:*

1. **DO NOT NAP DURING THE DAY.** You may feel

refreshed, but it could make it harder to get to sleep or stay asleep during the 1st part of the night. You should always look for the *reason* you cannot stay awake all day. Saying 'I enjoy my nap' is not a good enough *reason*. There is a difference between the word *reason* (an explanation) and the word *excuse* (to overlook). Needing to nap is an excuse for not being healthy enough to stay awake. The *reason* you nap is based on the weakness in your total health.

2. **KEEP YOUR SINUSES OPEN.** If you snore, you … *or anyone near you* … cannot sleep deep enough for healing. You will not snore if you breathe through your nose. But, if your sinus is blocked, you will breathe through your mouth … **and snore.** *Use a good nose spray with two sprays in each nose, sniffing hard after each spray; then sniffing hard through both nostrils, and blow if needed. This must be done three times a day until snoring stops.* Check your health food store for nasal spray options such as Xlear nose spray.

3. **EXERCISE DAILY.** The simple truth is you need to make your body tired enough to want to sleep. Exercise moves the toxic wastes out of your body that interfere with healthy body function. Isometric exercises flex and hold muscles for a short period of time to help leverage the relaxation impulse. YOU CANNOT TRY TO FALL ASLEEP! RELAX AND ALLOW SLEEP TO FIND YOU … try this:

    i. Lie on your back, inhale through your nose and exhale slowly … **continue this routine throughout the routine.**

    ii. Tense your toes tightly for a count of 10 … relax.

    iii. Tense your calves, count to 10 … relax. Continue to tense for a count of 10 and relax each of the following: thighs, buttocks, stomach, hands, arms, shoulders, neck and face.

    iv. Finally tighten all muscles for a count of 10 and relax. Repeat routine if you are not relaxed enough to sleep.

4. **CHANGE YOUR DIET.** Sugary snacks before bedtime may at first give you energy, but when your blood sugar drops you get sleepy. When it drops even lower during the night you wake up and cannot get back to sleep. Food allergies can wake you up during the night as your body starts to withdraw from the food. It is worth a try to consider food allergies as the cause of an early morning wake-up call you would rather not have. Generally considered high allergenic foods include corn, milk, beef, soy, peanut and gluten grains like wheat, oats, rye, spelt and barley. Caffeine products may also have to be evaluated. Some people can have sleep problems if they consume caffeine products in the late afternoon or later … even healthy green tea. Alcohol puts some people to sleep and energizes other people. *Learn how food or drink affects you.* **AVOID THE AMOUNT OF LIQUID BEFORE BEDTIME THAT MAKES YOU GO TO THE BATHROOM BEFORE 4 AM.** Do not drink any water 3 hours before going to bed, except a small amount if needed for bedtime supplements or medications.

5. **IMPROVE DIGESTION.** This helps to make hormones that control all bodily functions, including sleep hormones. *Digestion helps you support your ability to produce fuel for energy instead of converting nutrients to fat. THE ONLY WAY YOU KNOW IF YOU ARE DIGESTING WELL IS WITH THE SALIVA PH TEST THAT SHOULD BE BETWEEN 6.6 AND NO HIGHER THAN 7.2.*

6. **YOUR BEDROOM SHOULD HAVE STRICT RULES.** The night-light should be in the bathroom or hallway and not in the bedroom. Light in the bedroom stops the production of sleep hormones. You should reserve your dark, cool bedroom for sleep and intimacy. Your bedroom

should not be a place of work or watching scary movies or news. **TURN OFF ELECTRICAL APPLIANCES.** Do not sleep with a computer or TV on (best unplugged if not in use) or any other electrical appliance near your bed like electric clocks (use battery clocks), charging bases with cordless phones or cell phone chargers. **SELECT A COMFORTABLE ROOM TEMPERATURE** that is not too hot or too cold. Do not select too few covers or too many as an uncomfortable temperature interrupts sleep.

7. **YOU NEED PLENTY OF BRIGHT FULL SPECTRUM LIGHT IF YOU ARE INDOORS MOST OF THE DAY.** These are not ordinary fluorescent bulbs or regular light bulbs. Full spectrum lights mimic daylight that contributes to melatonin production you will need at night to help you sleep.

8. **USE ONLY NATURAL FIBER BEDDING AND SLEEPWEAR.** The quality of your bed can make a huge difference in restful sleep. A typical *chemically manufactured* mattress is made primarily from crude oil and natural gas derivatives: polyurethane, Styrofoam, polyester, dyes, fire retardants and a host of other chemicals. Polyurethane foam, as an example, is made from a number of ingredients that are recognized carcinogens. **New 'technologically advanced' chemically manufactured bedding and synthetic sleepwear are health disasters!!!!** *No wonder the typical American getting so little rest at night has an immune system that is wiped out.* **I suggest you cover your mattress and your pillow with an organic barrier cloth cover you can order from 1-800-Janices, or other natural product catalogs you can find on Google. WASH NATURAL FIBER BEDDING AND SLEEPWEAR BEFORE USING.** The formaldehyde sizing in 100% cotton needs to be washed out unless it says organic cotton; formaldehyde will not wash out in perma-press cotton. Use only natural laundry products and avoid synthetic fabric softeners and

fragrances. **Don't ask your body to work all night dealing with chemicals … you need your rest!!!**

9. **SHOWER OR BATHE** after dinner to get rid of dead skin cells that feed dust mites. Showering or bathing also clears negative frequencies for a more tranquil balance. There are calming herbal formulas that can be used in the bath or as a shower gel for relaxation. If you are too tired to shower at bedtime, or it wakes you up, then shower just before or after the evening meal. Dust mites live in pillows, mattresses, duvets and blankets where they lay their eggs and multiply. They are fed by a constant supply of dead skin cells off your body and get their water from your perspiration. The tiny mite droppings are made airborne by our slightest movement in bed. It is when the allergen is airborne that it can be harmful. When the allergen is inhaled or comes into contact with your skin, symptoms like asthma, eczema and other related allergic conditions can be triggered. Sooooooo … *you do not have to tell me twice to shower or bathe at night with a good brisk rub-down to get rid of skin cells that give mites dinner, wash my sheets weekly and the rest of the bedding monthly plus cover my mattress and pillows with barrier cloth.* I told my husband at our wedding ceremony he should say he would love me, respect me and shower at night. You can get bath and shower filters from www.gaiam.com.

10. **MOLD SENSITIVITY REQUIRES MORE FREQUENT LAUNDERING.** If you perspire a lot at night you may need to change your sheets two times a week and the pillow cases nightly. Mold grows on your pillowcase in 24 hours.

11. **CONSIDER SOFT MUSIC IN YOUR BEDROOM** while you are getting ready for bed. Listening to soothing music can help you sleep longer, wake up less frequently and be more awake during the day. Buy a tape recorder that shuts off at the end of the tape. *Listening to soft music that is*

so low you can hardly hear it every night often improves your sleep. Make sure the automatic shut off on the tape player is not so loud it wakes you up as it clicks off.

12. **TAKE THE RIGHT MINERALS AT BEDTIME.** Many people take calcium at bedtime, but for some people that can actually contribute to anxiety and cause muscles to contract. A better mineral to take is magnesium. Taking magnesium citrate powder at bedtime relieves anxiety and relaxes muscles. It also may increase bowel movements which is great for constipation but not good if your bowels tend to be loose … so consider your history and elimination needs before taking magnesium citrate (available in most health food stores).

13. **KEEP PETS OFF THE BED** to reduce parasites and mites in the bedding. You should not allow animals to wake you up every night when you need your valuable anti-aging sleep … *sorry.* Pets can be trained, so you decide who is training who!!! I trained my cat not to get on the bed and not to meow until I got up … honest!!! You can love your pets and give them a wonderful life without them robbing you of your health … *but they need to be trained just like children.* If keeping your dog or cat off your bed is unthinkable, at least consider ordering the Dog Proof Comforter from Orvis 1-800-541-3541 or orvis.com … then teach your pet to stay on the comforter.

14. **HOMEOPATHICS** that are *sold in many health food stores* calm and encourage deep sleep without a morning hangover. Homeopathic single ingredient or formulas are safe every night without concern about addiction and is the safest choice if you take prescription drugs. Do not take herbal sedatives with over-the-counter or prescription drugs without checking with your doctor first.

15. **BREAKING A BAD SLEEP PATTERN** can be difficult, but ***reprogramming your subconscious every night that you***

will sleep better, instead of going to bed confirming that you never sleep well is a critical place to start. Reprogramming the subconscious takes time, so do not give up just because you had your usual night. Do not get into the habit of staying up to read or watch TV if you cannot sleep. *Stay in bed, do the relaxation technique, keep your eyes close and at least rest.* It can take months of doing everything right to break a bad sleep pattern.

16. *TOO MUCH OF A GOOD THING DOES NOT MAKE IT BETTER!!! Do not stay in bed more than 8 hours, or you will lose calcium needed to balance pH.* This was proven with astronauts who lost calcium in weightlessness regardless of the amount of calcium they were given.

17. Sometimes a couple very much in love just cannot get needed sleep in the same bedroom. You can love your spouse dearly, find the right time for intimacy and choose to get your needed sleep in separate bedrooms. It should not be a sign that the honeymoon is over if you sleep apart. Some couples have a struggle sleeping if one is a bed hog and the other hangs on to the edge just trying to stay in bed. Some people hog the covers and leave the other chilly all night. Some people are light sleepers and cannot get back to sleep if the other gets up to the bathroom. Some people lay in bed for hours trying to get to sleep while the other reads or watches TV. Some people have tried everything and still snore making it very hard for the other to sleep. Some people do not sleep without tossing and turning all night, and can even hit the other and wake them up in a fretful turn. Some people like to go to bed clean but the other has an odor and prefers to shower in the morning. Some people cannot go back to sleep after the other gets up early each day to go to work … or comes in late from work. Some people like to sleep with a pet but the other objects to the pet's early morning needs that disturb sleep. WHATEVER THE REASON YOU SHOULD **FIRST** FIND A WAY

TO HAVE A RESTFUL NIGHTS SLEEP SO YOU CAN BE YOUR LOVING, BEST PERSONALITY THE NEXT DAY ... AND SAVE THE QUALITY OF YOUR RELATIONSHIP! Becoming moody and irritable from lack of sleep can make it easier for a person to make poor choices the next day. **One person may have spent so many years compromising good sleep they do not associate the daytime addictions to sleep deprivation.**

Resting the immune system from working all night is top priority as you try to survive all the stresses of living in modern America! Control your overall health to control your weight!!!

GOODNIGHT *zzzzzzzzzzzzzzzzzzz*

WEIGHT LOSS TIP # 6

CONSTIPATION

This clearly is no fun!!! Besides the discomfort, you can get very tired from retaining toxic wastes, your skin can break out, headaches often occur and you hesitate to put more food in when nothing is coming out. Your stomach bloats, body odor increases, **you gain weight** … *well, you get the picture.* The bowel is your sewage system of your body. *By abuse and neglect, the bowel can become dangerously foul!!!* Information on symptoms arising primarily from intestinal toxemia has filled volumes. Here are some user friendly recommendations that are **not intended to replace medical attention if needed:**

1. The NUMBER ONE cause of constipation is *NOT ENOUGH WATER!!!*

2. The NUMBER TWO cause of constipation is *NOT ENOUGH EXERCISE!!!*

3. The NUMBER THREE cause of constipation is *pH IMBALANCE!!!*

4. The NUMBER FOUR cause of constipation is *NOT ENOUGH GOOD BACTERIA* and increased bad microorganisms like Candida yeast or parasites!!!

5. The NUMBER FIVE cause of constipation is NOT ENOUGH FIBER AND TOO MUCH REFINED AND PROCESSED FOOD!!!

6. **The NUMBER SIX cause of constipation is** *POOR STRESS MANAGEMENT!!!*

Your colon is not meant to be a stainless steel holding tank for food. The colon can hold eight or more meals worth of undigested food and waste when you consume the typical American diet of refined and processed food. However, with an adequate fiber diet, enough water and exercise the colon holds about three meals. *It does not take a rocket scientist to figure out good elimination helps in weight control.*

Africans, with their high-fiber vegetable diet and large, moist uniformed stools have little hospital huts. Many constipated Americans with their red meat, white bread and small tubular stools end up in multi-story hospitals. Americans are quick to turn to laxatives but that can be addictive. There are many herbal laxative formulas in the health food stores that are gentle and *encourage support of the whole digestive-intestinal interrelated system.*

You will not get away with ignoring constipation. **DO NOT BE SATISFIED WITH LESS ELIMINATION THAN IS NEEDED TO PROTECT YOUR LIFE!!!** *GREAT … WHAT DOES THAT MEAN?* **THAT MEANS A LARGE MOVEMENT BEFORE NOON THAT IS EASY TO PASS AND 1-2 SMALLER ONES DURING THE DAY** (sorry … reading material in the bathroom should not be necessary). *The following non-laxative recommendations help most people:*

1. **Magnesium** is always low when constipated and should be the *1st line of defense to improve the problem.* Check with your health food store for product options to take at bedtime like magnesium citrate powder.

2. Some people need more help, so consider adding a **buffered Vitamin C powder** to the magnesium at bedtime. Too much magnesium can imbalance calcium so if a scoop of magnesium citrate powder is not enough to give you the elimination you want then you would be better to increase the Vitamin C until results are achieved.

3. Most people forget the obvious … **drink more water!**

4. Most people forget the obvious … **daily exercise!**

5. Most people do not know what their **pH balance** is so they do not know if their bowel is out of balance. *Get your pH paper and test yourself.*

6. Most people with constipation are low in **good bowel bacteria**. *Your best friend could be a dairy free probiotic supplement to replace needed good bacteria. Consider 2 daily, ½ hour before breakfast, LIFETIME!* This is especially important if you have old mercury fillings in your mouth, as mercury kills the good bacteria needed for a healthy bowel. Also, stress kills good bacteria … good luck not having stress living in modern America.

7. **A relaxing defecation schedule** is critical. Do not set the morning alarm so late that you have to rush. Because the circadian rhythm cycle for elimination ends at 12 noon, you can create body imbalances if your main elimination is later in the day. Some people will not eliminate until the next day if they miss that cycle.

8. **Eating organic food** is vital in your effort to have a healthy intestinal system. Our health statistics, including overweight, have changed drastically in the past 50 years when chemicals invaded every element of our lifestyle.

9. **Stress management** is a complicated subject that must be understood if you are going to control your digestive and elimination systems … *and thus control your health and weight.* There are three basic types of people … which one are you?

   STAGNATOR – do nothing about your health or slow weight gain over the years, and believe symptoms are all part of aging, giving birth, an accident etc., etc.

REACTOR – only worry when your health situation gets out of hand, or one day your weight becomes unacceptable.

PROACTOR – living the good life with a healthy body and mind because you understand and practice the **laws of wellness** … obviously this should be your goal.

*"The natural healing force within us is the
greatest force in getting well."*

-Hippocrates, Father of Medicine

WEIGHT LOSS TIP # 7

PROBIOTICS

THE *ONLY WAY TO GOOD HEALTH IS THROUGH THE DIGESTIVE SYSTEM*

The typical American society favors the wrong kinds of liquid, overeating, eating hard to digest proteins, eating wrong combinations of foods and eating under physical and emotional stress. WE CANNOT TAKE FOR GRANTED THAT THE PRESENT EATING PRACTICES OF MANY AMERICANS ARE ACCEPTABLE FOR THE PROMOTION OF HEALTH AND WEIGHT CONTROL. *WHAT WE HAVE IS A SOCIETY OF ACUTE AND CHRONICALLY ILL, WEAK AND OVERWEIGHT PEOPLE.* THERE IS A LOT MORE TO WEIGHT LOSS THAN CALORIE COUNTING AND MEASURING YOUR FOOD!!! **THERE IS A LOT MORE TO *MAINTAINING* WEIGHT LOSS THAN CALORIE COUNTING AND MEASURING YOUR FOOD!!!**

Research has discovered that the one thing healthy people have in common is a high level of 'friendly' bacteria throughout their digestive system. Antibiotics given as prescription drugs and antibiotics in food destroy this *friendly* intestinal micro-flora. Some of the other offenders that can deplete *friendly* flora are stress, alcohol, sugar, drugs, processed foods, tobacco smoke, high estrogen levels, chlorinated tap water and even the aging process. The opposite of antibiotics that kill both illness causing bacteria **AND** friendly flora, is probiotics which literally means 'promoting life'. Probiotics promote good digestion and other beneficial functions listed below that make them essential to life. ***Most people do*** *not understand the power of these tiny life savers in their search for wellness and weight control.*

In the early 1900's the probiotics theory by Russian Nobel Prize winner Elie Metchnikoff concluded that the long life of Bulgarian peasants was the result of their daily consumption of fermented milk products. It is this lactobacillus acidophilus that points to the health and longevity of many cultures. Metchnikoff believed that the bacillus that fermented the milk positively influenced the *friendly* micro-flora of the colon, thereby decreasing the toxic effects of *unfriendly* bacteria. *One hundred years ago we were not all reacting to milk in the same way we are today. The daily challenged immune system of most Americans is a lot different than in the days of Daniel Boone. This too often challenged immune system plus the increased use of beef and dairy products has changed the tolerance level of these foods for many people from babies to seniors.* So, we should get our *friendly* cultures from another yogurt source. We tend to have a society high in estrogen due to the estrogen look-a-likes in chemicals. The high use of soy that also has estrogen look-a-likes makes soy a questionable yogurt alternative … look for easy to digest goat or sheep yogurt. The commercial yogurt processing today is not the same quality yogurt that people used to eat. Modern day commercial yogurt may not have enough good bacteria to produce colony growth. To set up good colony growth of *friendly* bacteria, you need **strong probiotics taken on an empty stomach first thing in the morning 30 minutes before breakfast … everyday.**

WHAT ARE SOME OF THE BENEFITS OF PROBIOTICS?

- They provide the **balance** to control all unwanted microorganisms, including parasites and Candida yeast that grow in the absence of healthy micro-flora. These unwanted organisms eat up the nutrients your body needs to support health and normal weight.

- They **normalize bowel movements** to control both constipation and diarrhea.

- They stimulate the formation of antibodies to **improve immune function** and allergy control.

- They create at least 7 essential **B vitamins** necessary for stress management and digestion.

- They assist in the **digestion of dairy products**. People who get diarrhea from poor digestion of milk sugar are low in probiotics.

- They help **regulate the entire digestive system** controlling abnormalities in the intestines that can lead to many skin disorders.

- They help **regulate cholesterol** levels in the blood.

- They help **regulate hormone levels** that can mellow your day making you more likely to make better choices for general health and weight control!

- They help **eliminate intestinal gas**, bloating and other signs of indigestion.

*So run ... **do not walk** to your health food store, and purchase the highest quality, strongest, dairy and beef free broad spectrum vegetarian probiotic supplement you can find.* **YOUR WHOLE SLIMMER BODY WILL LOVE YOU FOR IT!!!**

WEIGHT LOSS TIP # 8

ORGANIC FOOD AND PRODUCTS

Now it is time to go shopping for food and products. You do not have to throw out hundreds of dollars worth of purchases, but you should know that you can improve your energy through your **correct choice of new purchases**.

The typical American diet is disease producing. We must stop pouring chemicals into our bodies with herbicides, pesticides and fungicides in chemically raised produce, hormones and antibiotics in animal products and a multitude of chemicals in processed and refined food. **ORGANIC FOOD IS A CRITICAL CONSIDERATION IN YOUR WEIGHT LOSS PLAN.** *Nutrition through healthy organic food is not the whole health and weight loss story, but it is something for which there is no substitute.* An organic diet sets up the process of building health and energy. Commercial food can be grown with only water plus added nitrogen, potassium, and phosphorus. The rest of the minerals, as well as some trace minerals can be missing in some farmland; and added herbicides, pesticides and round-up chemicals produce toxic wastes that can be disease producing.

The most difficult part of any dietary change is a person's ATTITUDE. The key to dietary change is *emphasizing* how many delicious and healthy foods are available … *NOT* what you have to give up! *Because you choose to be healthy, you can choose to reduce consumption of unhealthy choices, find acceptable substitutes when possible and treat yourself occasionally to foods you miss socially.* How you react to those foods will determine how 'social' you are willing to be. The reward for dietary changes may be the desire for energy and weight loss that you are seeking. Don't set yourself up to feel frustrated because you WANT something you now know is not good for you. **Once you start to feel better, have more energy and start losing weight, you will realize the importance of eating to live, rather than living to eat.** *Trust me; I was seriously ill for 20 years, so being healthy is a real kick!!!!* I travel a lot, eat out at least one time a week and enjoy a piece of coconut cake for my birthday (that I sometimes make organic at home). The difference is that I am **SELECTIVE** of what I eat out … and **what I eat at home is always organic or all natural!!!** I make healthy cookies, muffins, even fudge and desserts with low glycemic ingredients, gluten free grains, and a dash of love.

Pesticides include insecticides, herbicides and fungicides. Farmers use billions of pounds of pesticides every year, and many have been found by the *U.S. Environmental Protection Agency (EPA)* to be carcinogenic. The EPA has registered close to 900 pesticides, which are formulated into thousands of products according to the *Northwest Coalition for Alternatives to Pesticides.* One pesticide classification used in agriculture, called organochlorines, acts like estrogen and has been linked to breast cancer. *The Lancet* December 1999 found a correlation between exposure to organochlorines and pancreatic cancer (on the rise for the first time in history). In her book, *Chemical Sensitivities*, Dr. Sherry Rogers explains that when pesticides **break down**, they produce substances called 'metabolites' that are *more toxic than the original toxins used to kill pests.* Studies by the *National Academy of Sciences* and the *Environmental Working Group* found that children exposed to carcinogenic pesticides are at a higher risk of future cancer.

You must first understand the problem to appreciate why organic food is a no-brainer! Organic food does not only eliminate dangerous chemicals, but it also eliminates genetically engineered food. GE foods are engineered to tolerate heavier doses of chemicals. The first large-scale commercial harvest of GE crops in the US happened in 1996. By 1999, one-fourth of American crops were genetically engineered. Unlabelled GE foods now account for as much as two-thirds of all foods … and more are on the way. Since these foods have been rushed to the market so quickly, scientists remain in the dark about the long-term impacts of GE foods on our health. ***Organic does mean it is not genetically engineered or genetically modified food,*** **but a label that states it is not genetically engineered or genetically modified does not mean it is organic.**

The organic food industry is growing every year, and many regular supermarkets now carry organic products. We use more chemicals in our food industry than any other country in the world, so imported food items from Europe may not state organic but may be raised with those standards. *Except for imported food, or canned fish, every food item in my kitchen is certified organic or all natural.* The only time I eat non-organic food is in a restaurant. **These common titles you will see in different health food stores are all environmentally friendly and include:**

- **USDA Certified Organic** means the land has not been treated with any toxic materials or chemical fertilizers for 3 years.

- **Local Non-Certified** usually comes from farmers who practice organic farming methods but for meaningful reasons have chosen not to be certified.

- **Biologically Grown** produce is grown by developing the natural fertility of the soil, avoiding use of artificial fertilizers and chemical sprays.

- **Integrated Pest Management** (IPM) is socially acceptable, environmentally responsible and economically practical crop protection. They resort to chemicals only if pests reach economically damaging levels.

Some chain health food stores intermingle organic produce with non-organic, and that is confusing to the shopper new to healthier eating. Since some produce stockers may not always change the label when current deliveries change from organic to non-organic, you can only be sure it is organic if it has a certified organic label as a sticker or twisty. I prefer to shop at health food stores that only sell organic or environmentally friendly produce. ***We are paying a huge price for fooling with Mother Nature.***

If scientists are experimenting through genetic engineering to grow fish at four times the natural rate … what is the risk to you? Eat only ocean fish or seafood, not farm raised Atlantic salmon, tilapia, trout, bluefish, rockfish or catfish. Some health food stores sell ecologically safe farm raised fish and seafood. **We will have to take a hard look at a lot of our so called *new and improved* ideas to find a way to turn around the shocking poor health and overweight statistics in this country.**

I do not eat cow dairy products, beef, deep fried food, processed food or soy products. I eat buffalo, lamb or duck and organic turkey bacon or sausage. Fowl products are all organic, and I order ocean fish or seafood in a restaurant (no farm raised fish unless there is no better choice on the menu). I eat ocean or ecologically farm raised fish at home, no alcohol or caffeine, organic low fructose fruit choices no more than once a day (discussed in Tip #12), and only non-dairy rice milk. My dairy needs are met with Manchego sheep cheese and Water Buffalo mozzarella, also sheep yogurt. Refined sugar is limited to special occasions outside of my home and at home I use only Stevia or Coconut Secret products. Of course I eat lots of organic vegetables, organic nuts and seeds, organic sprouted flaxseed, rice pastas, super digestible gluten free Quinoa, Teff and Millet. *I was born on February 3, 1934 and look many years younger, with a 5 foot 2 inch frame that stays slim. I have energy that lasts all day, a desire to be in service to mankind, and a joyful enthusiasm for life … you decide what you want to eat.*

Not all references to being sensitive mean mental or emotional. There are biological explanations for other kinds of sensitivities. Some people with hyperactive nervous systems react stronger to chemicals than others. We **BELIEVE** we tolerate toxins in the air we breathe, the water we drink, the food we eat, the chemically based clothing we wear and the chemicals in the household products we use. *If you **suddenly** become sensitive to an exposure you thought was previously tolerated, it could be a warning sign that your digestive, elimination, circulatory and immune systems have been **weakened for too long.*** Every day you come in contact with toxins from chemical products that you've used for years, and you may not think to blame an old favorite on your recent change of health. A build up of toxic chemicals can produce any chronic symptom that the doctors cannot trace back to a definite cause. *Rather than frantically trying the latest advertised 'detox' product, **first reduce your exposure to the toxins in everyday products you use.*** SPEND MORE TIME FINDING WAYS NOT TO PUT TOXIC WASTES INTO YOUR BODY AND LESS TIME TRYING TO FIGURE OUT WAYS TO GET THOSE TOXIC WASTES OUT!!!

I purchase all natural household and personal care products. Stores and catalogs that carry natural products are constantly growing. We all want to kill ants, but by attacking **their** nervous system, you may be attacking your own. My personal disaster story occurred when my husband told our pest control man about a bug problem in our master bathroom. Without discussing it with us first, he put a product behind a plant and the toilet, so we remained unaware. In about a week I lost control of my neck muscles and could hardly swallow. I struggled with a weak throat and hoarse voice for months even after we located the problem and removed the product. Needless to say, we called the company and they are never allowed inside our home again. I wrote a newspaper article about using sugar and yeast to kill ants instead of dangerous chemicals and they misquoted me saying, *"Dori hates white sugar, and she says let the black ants eat it."* **We do not need bad journalism in this country, but we do need a major reality check on the connection between our obsession with chemicals and the development of disease.** You can check the internet for healthy options to killing pests. STOP BUYING PRODUCTS THAT STATE *"DANGER", "WARNING"* OR *"CAUTION"* ON THE LABEL.

BE A HEALTHY CONSUMER AND LET THE STORES KNOW WHAT YOU WANT TO BUY!!! YOU CAN MAKE A BIG DIFFERENCE THROUGH YOUR PURCHASING CHOICES! MONEY TALKS IN THIS COUNTRY … AND YOU HAVE A VOICE. BUY ITEMS THAT SAY USDA CERTIFIED ORGANIC … ALL NATURAL … OR ECOLOGICALLY FRIENDLY!!! YOUR ADRENAL GLANDS ARE WEAKENED BY CHEMICALS, AND THEY ARE NEEDED FOR MORE IMPORTANT WORK … LIKE BODY FUNCTIONS THAT CONTROL YOUR WEIGHT!!!

MINERAL DEFICIENCIES

How many times have you said (or heard an overweight person say), *"I eat too much when I'm angry … or upset … or frustrated?" Maybe the* *statement is, "When I'm too tired I get irritable and all my will power* *goes down the tube." There are many comments that apply here but they* *are all excuses … not reasons.* **We too often make excuses for our own** **behavior … or others, without accepting responsibility for choices** **that may have contributed to the mental or emotional state.**

Politics and the big business of disease have led Americans down *a challenging path.* **TOO OFTEN THE AMERICAN DREAM** **CAN BECOME THE AMERICAN POOR HEALTH AND** **OVERWEIGHT NIGHTMARE.** We need to **wake up** and realize that what we are doing **IS NOT WORKING!** *The direction towards* *health education instead of only the treatment of disease is getting better.* *However, many health tips that are given to the general public are too* *few, too late for many, too incomplete and too fragmented to support the* *body as a whole and be of lasting value.* We blame our frustrations on the wrong things because of our national standards. *No one seems to* *know how to stop the runaway train.* **Never before in the history of the** **world has there been a greater need for health recommendations that** **SIMPLY WORK!** *Health is simple … it is disease that is so complicated!* *In disease weight gain is easy.*

We have to stop kidding ourselves that the food we put into our mouths contains all the nutrients we see listed in the food charts. Commercial farming, processing, refining, shipping, storage, additives, microwaving or cooking all contribute to nutritionally deficient meals. **JUST BECAUSE YOU ARE NOT HUNGRY DOES NOT MEAN YOUR CELLS ARE WELL FED!!!** To get the most nutrients from your very important mealtime be aware that:

- Organic fresh is best if it is really fresh and not wilted.

- Organic dried is next best because low heat does not destroy nutrients and enzymes like high heat. Be aware that mold may be a problem with dried food if you are severely mold sensitive.

- Organic frozen food is next best, but may be better than fresh if you live far from a health food store and cannot shop weekly to replace fresh food.

- Organic canned food is least nutritious unless you drink all the liquid that contains valuable minerals. If you have an excess of organic food from your garden you will preserve more food value if you dry or freeze.

People can easily be fooled when it comes to the actual nutrition of what they eat, as this story about canned peas describes:

> *Plants cannot take up nutrients that are not available in the soil, so a crop of peas grown commercially today may not have the same nutritional quality as peas grown a hundred years ago. Nutrients are further lost in transportation and washing. When the peas are canned, minerals are lost in the water and some vitamins are affected in various degrees. Heat destroys ALL enzymes to assist in digestion, so your body must do all the work. Storage and distribution vary, but the canned peas could be several years old when you decide to cook them for dinner. Then you boil the peas and throw the mineral-rich water down the drain, so your unhealthy hydrogenated margarine will stick to them. After the farmer, the packer, the grocer, and you have done your best to eliminate a*

> *shocking percentage of nutrition from those peas, you take comfort in having eaten your vegetable for dinner.*

One of my favorite research books has been **THE CHEMISTRY OF MAN** by Bernard Jensen., Ph.D. In over 50 years of work Dr. Jensen watched patients recover and thrive when their diets were adjusted to provide the chemical elements their bodies needed. **HOW SIMPLE IS THAT!!!** Dr. Jenson's research showed some of the mental and emotional symptoms that can be caused by **simple mineral deficiencies. People struggling with weight gain will see themselves in one or more of the following low minerals:**

- **CALCIUM** (the "knitter") – memory reduction, antisocial conduct, impatience, apprehension.

- **CARBON** (the "builder") – unfeeling, bitter, unfriendly, overcritical, poor judgment.

- **CHLORINE** (the "cleanser") – gloom, low self-esteem or spirit, everything out of balance.

- **FLUORINE** (the anti-resistant element) – awkward and vulgar but person convinced he/she is polished and graceful, false confidence.

- **HYDROGEN** (the "moisturizer") – difficult to please, temperamental, intolerant.

- **IODINE** (the "metabolizer") – tired, depressed, frustrated, un-balanced emotions.

- **IRON** (the "frisky horse") – self-pity, antisocial, memory deficient, nervous stress, short temper.

- **MAGNESIUM** (the "relaxer") – hyperactive, nervous personality, moods not grounded, life seems uninteresting.

- **MANGANESE** (the "love" element) – mental confusion, quarrelsomeness, impatience, unstable.

- **NITROGEN** (the "restrainer") – hypochondriac with every ache exaggerated, mind is changeable, focus on extremes with nothing in the middle.

- **OXYGEN** (the "giver of life") – nervous, emotional instability, stubborn, hypersensitivity, secretive, ill-tempered.

- **PHOSPHORUS** (the "light bearer") – self-pity, morbidity, hypersensitivity, craves affection but self-conscious.

- **POTASSIUM** (the "great alkalizer") – fears, changeable moods, mostly negative, low drive.

- **SILICON** (the "magnetic element") – depression, mental strain, brooding, hopeless, argumentative and ungratified.

- **SULFUR** (the "heating element") – irritability, worry, stormy emotions, impulsive.

- **SODIUM** (the "youth element") – mental confusion, mental exhaustion, quarrelsome, dull, disinterested, depressed.

THE SOLUTION TO SUPPORTING POSITIVE THOUGHTS THAT ENCOURAGE MAKING POSITIVE CHOICES IS SIMPLE ... PUT NUTRITIONAL ENERGY INTO YOUR BODY INSTEAD OF DEPLETING YOUR BODY OF ENERGY WITH POOR DIETARY CHOICES. SO HOW DO YOU DO THAT? READ THIS BOOK AND THEN READ IT AGAIN!!!

If you think the recommendations in this book do not sound simple, consider the health complications of being overweight ... of having unnecessary stressful family issues that challenge or destroy the family unit ... or straining the family budget with challenging expenses ... or having a serious disease ... or losing the quality of life ... or life itself far too soon. *All changes in your normal routine take time and determination to become your new routine, and any effort you put in will produce rewards.* If you are not happy with your present state of wellness or your present weight, then do not keep doing what you have been doing because it is easy and familiar … **DO SOMETHING DIFFERENT … AND MAKE A DIFFERENCE THAT YOU CAN LIVE WITH IN A WAY THAT MAKES LIFE JOYFUL!!!**

We are a well fed and still malnourished society, so a good sentence to start with is, **"IF IT IS NEW AND IMPROVED, FORGET IT."** Only organic, unprocessed food can give you the full quota of vitamins and minerals in a state that your body can effectively use.

WEIGHT LOSS TIP #10

NIGHTSHADE FOODS

You may have never heard of the nightshade word and not at all sure what it has to do with weight loss. I was watching an advertisement on TV and they said by 2018 over ½ of Americans will be overweight. Since so many people lose weight successfully on the usual weight loss programs … why do so many people gain it back? With all the attention to weight loss and many books by famous people being purchased by the millions … why is weight loss still such a problem? **IN MY OPINION IT IS BECAUSE THE EMPHASIS ON WEIGHT LOSS IS JUST THAT … WEIGHT LOSS. THE EMPHASIS IS NOT ON TOTAL WELLNESS.** Another reason is that every weight loss book seems to disagree as to how you accomplish weight loss. *This book intends to fill in all the information gaps missing from the usual approach to weight loss and make the program more individualized.* If your body is under stress or pain for any reason, it can make your effort to lose weight more complicated… even unsuccessful.

A person trying to deal with the details of weight loss does not want to also deal with pain. If you have joint pain anywhere, your body is shouting that you have an inflammation. **The first line of defense is water** because every joint in the body is cushioned with water. Toxic wastes from poor digestion due to dehydration can irritate joints. Make sure your saliva pH is in the 6.6 - 7.0 range for good digestion. Many people try in vain using a multitude of joint supplements that may help some people … **but this is not dealing with the CAUSE.** Long term unresolved inflammation will damage tissues and lead to other problems

… like sabotaging your weight loss effort because it is too painful to walk or exercise.

Joints can be a target for allergic reactions to foods, so **the second line of defense** is to stop all cow dairy and beef products, as well as gluten grains (wheat, oats, rye, barley, spelt, and for some people also non-grain buckwheat). Where there is inflammation, your body produces extra white blood cells to clean up the debris. *These extra cells make chemicals that can produce pain, so the more you eat the food that triggers this response, the more pain you have.*

The **nightshade family of foods** can often produce pain *chemicals* in people with joint symptoms. These chemicals react differently than an allergic response. People love foods in this family, and these foods can produce a physiological addiction because they contain small quantities of powerful drug-like substances called alkaloids. Even a small amount of a nightshade food can cause severe joint pain in some people. If you have any joint pain, consider a trial 100% elimination diet for at least one month. This trial will be more successful if you eat at home and not in a restaurant. If you get any relief from the joint pain at all, continue for another two to three months to allow the area to settle down before you attempt a test meal from the list of foods below. *Some people can have these foods occasionally in small amounts after the body has healed from the acute stage of inflammation.* **During a one month test period** *completely* **eliminate the following foods:**

Red and white potatoes	Tomatoes	All peppers
Potato starch	Paprika	Curry
Cayenne pepper	Chile	Eggplant

Tobacco is also from the nightshade family so evaluate this exposure if you smoke or are around smokers. It is very easy to get these foods in complex processed products with multiple ingredients, so eating food you prepare yourself is a good plan. *All gluten free products will use potato starch that may be referred to as modified food starch, modified vegetable protein, modified vegetable starch and hydrolyzed vegetable protein.* Deep fried food in a restaurant may be cooked in the same oil as French fried potatoes. Potato starch is frequently the filler in prescription and over-the-counter medications. If you are very sensitive you can have a compounding pharmacy make a prescription using rice filler. Vodka is made from fermented potatoes.

Why is this important? **BECAUSE IN YOUR QUEST FOR WELLNESS YOU WILL BE MORE SUCCESSFUL IN ALL YOUR EFFORTS ... INCLUDING A WEIGHT LOSS PROGRAM ... IF YOU ARE NOT DEALING WITH HIDDEN ISSUES THAT STRESS YOUR BODY.**

WEIGHT LOSS TIP #11

SALICYLATE FOODS

One of the problems I have with many of the weight loss recipes is the *lack of dealing with individual problems*. **FOCUSING JUST ON WEIGHT LOSS MAY BE THE BEST WAY TO SABOTAGE THE LONG TERM SUCCESS OF YOUR EFFORT!** Just like the nightshade foods can be a problem for some people dealing with joint pain, salicylate foods can be a problem for some people dealing with chemical sensitivities. Many hyperactive children become nervous, anxious adults because they *never* dealt with the foods that affected them chemically. *This anxiety leads to overeating … and you know the rest.*

Phenol is an organic compound obtained from coal tar. Phenol also occurs naturally in poison ivy, poison oak, thyme oil and some spring water in a natural coal area, plus all smoke. The chemical phenol is the starting point in many commercial products. *To make a complex subject simple, if you cannot tolerate smoke, traffic, road repair work, perfume, aspirin, artificial colors and flavors in processed foods or processed foods in general, you should look at phenol sensitivity as a **CAUSE** of your symptoms.* If you are sick and tired of being sick and tired and nothing you do medically improves the quality of your day, it could be the phenol based herbicides and pesticides in your non-organic food. **We have technologically advanced ourselves into a mess!!!**

The chemicals phenol and salicylate in food are molecularly the same in the body. This intolerance to the *build-up* of certain chemicals in the body is not the same as an allergic reaction. *Even if you rotated* *all the foods listed below that are in different biological families, you could still accumulate **daily** salicylate chemicals.* **The following foods contain salicylate chemicals:**

almonds	cherries	grapes, raisins, currants
apples	all berries	nectarines, tangerines
apricots	all oranges	cucumbers
peaches	tomatoes	green/red peppers
plums/prunes	cider and wine vinegar	rose hips
beer	aspirin	distilled drinks except vodka
wintergreen	mint	cloves
coffee	regular tea	coloring in food, drinks, and drugs
chili powder	soft drinks (except 7 UP in glass bottles)	peanuts with skin
cayenne	canned green and black olives	coconut oil
radish	chicory	alfalfa sprouts
artichoke	broccoli	eggplant
fresh spinach	sweet potato	green zucchini
olive oil	brazil nuts	macadamia nuts
pine nuts	pistachio nuts	sesame oil
walnut oil	all dried fruits	melons
grapefruit	kiwi fruit	avocado
mustard	black pepper	curry
cumin	ginger	honey
nutmeg	oregano	paprika
peppermint	rosemary	sage
Tabasco	tarragon	thyme
turmeric	white vinegar	Worcester sauce
bay leaf	pimento	cinnamon
blueberries	vanilla	pineapple
cranberries		

The following list may be a problem for the severely sensitive, or may be tolerated if eaten no more than twice a week on a four day rotation:

cinnamon	vanilla	white or red potato
carrots	banana	pineapple
blueberries	green peas	nonorganic cranberries

These foods do not contain salicylate chemicals:

All animal meat, fish, seafood and fowl; some stores have been caught coloring red meat to make it look fresher.

All non-dairy milk and non-dairy ice cream that does not contain salicylate ingredients listed above, Manchego sheep cheese, water buffalo mozzarella, plain goat or sheep yogurt.

All nuts & seeds, fats & oils not listed.

All pastas and all grains (watch some ingredients in prepared products).

All fruits and vegetables not listed above."

Herbal teas unless they contain ingredients listed above. 7-Up is the only carbonated drink allowed. All distilled drinks except vodka. Spearmint tea is free of salicylates.

Before you panic, even if your history suggests these foods are a problem, as you become healthier you may be able to rotate a few favorites on a four day rotation. *Giving up favorite foods and feeling better is worth more than wondering why you do not feel well and no one seems to be able to give you a reason.* **Giving up favorite foods and feeling better is worth more than losing weight and getting frustrated that you gained it all back.**

REMEMBER YOUR GOAL IS NOT JUST TO LOSE WEIGHT BUT TO FEEL BETTER AND KEEP THE WEIGHT OFF IN THE FUTURE! IF TRYING A HEALTHIER NEW

TWIST ON AN OLD RECIPE SOLVES THE SYMPTOMS THAT MESS UP YOUR DAY, CONSIDER THAT A REAL BONUS!!! LEARN TO EAT TO LIVE AND NOT LIVE TO EAT. KNOWLEDGE IS POWER IN YOUR EFFORT TO TAKE CONTROL OF YOUR LIFE ... YOUR HEALTH ... AND YOUR WEIGHT CONTROL.

LECTINS

A molecule that has been sabotaging the digestive health of millions of people every year is found in many foods and plants. This molecule is a protein called lectin that attaches itself to sugars naturally found in human cells. Lectins can mimic health problems such as headaches and brain fog, skin disorders, weight gain … or weight loss, bloating, fatigue, mucus buildup, digestive symptoms, joint pain, and symptoms of low immune response such as colds or flu.

Since lectins naturally attach to sugar molecules in the body they act like a magnet to those sugars. This is viewed by the body as invasive so the immune system sends white blood cells to the area and creates an inflammatory response. This inflammatory response can occur in any area of the body.

Lectins are found in most of the foods you eat, but are very high in gluten grains (wheat, barley, rye, oats and spelt), the nightshade foods (tomato, potato, pepper, eggplant, tobacco, curry), all legumes, all dairy, chicken and eggs. Eliminating any of the above foods that you LOVE and eat on a regular basis will help reduce some local inflammation.

Lectins are in many other foods you eat so it is not possible to eliminate all exposures to Lectin proteins. You can even be exposed to environmental lectins on your lawn, pollens from your garden and ingredients in medicines and cosmetics. For more information, you can contact 1-800-746-4513 or www.truehealth.com.

Now that you are totally concerned … what do you do? The best way to deal with lectins is to understand "The Laws of Wellness" that keep your digestion and immune system strong.

IMPROVING YOUR DIGESTIVE SYSTEM WITH CORRECT HYDRATION, ORGANIC FOOD AND A BALANCE pH IS THE FIRST STEP IN CONTROLLING YOUR BODY'S REACTION TO LECTINS. WHEN YOU ARE BASICALLY UNHEALTHY THE BODY REACTS IN A "PROTECTIVE" MODE AND CAUSES HAVOC (SYMPTOMS) IN THE ATTEMPT TO PROTECT YOU.

WEIGHT LOSS TIP #13

INSULIN RESISTANCE

Insulin is the leading actor in your health performance. The pancreas makes too much insulin when the diet is too high in simple carbohydrates (refined grains and pastas, sugar and desserts, fresh and dried fruit, fruit juice, fruit jams and jelly, products containing fruit, white potatoes, alcohol, sugar cured food and tobacco).

Cells in all parts of your body can become insulin resistant because they are trying to protect themselves from the toxic effects of high insulin. They protect themselves by down regulating their receptor activity and even a number of receptors to reduce the noxious stimuli all the time. It is like turning down the volume on irritating music … and that allows the beginning of disease to start.

LIVER

The liver is the first to become resistant and suppresses the production of sugar. The sugar in your circulation comes from sugar you eat and when needed, like in the morning, from the liver. Because of insulin resistance the liver does not release stored sugar at night thinking there is too much insulin so you wake up groggy. And then the liver releases a bunch of sugar to wake you up.

MUSCLES/STORED FAT

The next tissues to become resistant are the muscles that burn sugar with insulin. When resistant, the muscles do not burn the sugar and this can raise blood sugar levels. Fat cells are the last to become resistant so for a while your fat cells retain their sensitivity to insulin. Eventually as excess sugar is not burned as energy it is stored as fat and your weight goes up.

LINING OF THE ARTERIES

As major tissues become more insulin resistant, excess insulin causes plaque buildup in the circulatory system. Any cardiovascular disease could have its origin from insulin resistance. Insulin resistance is a precursor to diabetes and overweight people can head for not just diabetes, but heart disease as well.

DIET RECOMMENDATION

Eliminate all gluten grains, rice and corn.

Eliminate all fruit and fruit juices.

Eliminate all starchy vegetables like potatoes, sweet potatoes and legumes.

Eliminate all refined sugar, honey, agave and maple syrup.

Eliminate all refined sugary desserts except for social occasions.

The following foods are allowed unless eliminated for other reasons:

The following gluten free grains: quinoa, teff and millet.

All Coconut Secret products that include Coconut Aminos (a substitute for soy sauce), Coconut Nectar (a substitute for maple syrup, honey and agave), Coconut Vinegar (a substitute for grain or apple vinegar that may not be tolerated) and Coconut Crystals (substitute for sugar in any recipe).

All protein.

All nuts and seeds.

All cold pressed oils.

All salad dressings that do not contain sugar.

Spaghetti squash, butternut squash or any summer squash.

Tapioca made with non-sweetened milk, coconut lite or almond milk.

Consider the peanut butter and muffin recipes on the back of the Bob's Red Mill Teff bag. However, be sure to substitute the Coconut Nectar for the maple syrup in the cookies. Substitute the Coconut Crystals for the sugar, and quinoa flour for the rice flour in the muffins. Any recipe can be made with part quinoa, millet, coconut and teff flours in proportions as desired based on preference.

All non-starch vegetables. When in doubt, refer to www. glycemicindex.com. Type in a specific food to find its glycemic index and consider any food under 55.

WEIGHT LOSS TIP #14

FRUCTOSE

By now you may be afraid to read the next page for fear you will lose more foods you love. Remember ... ***not all people*** have a problem with the nightshade foods, and ***not all people*** have a problem with salicylate foods. **HOWEVER, ALL PEOPLE INCLUDING SKINNY PEOPLE HAVE A PROBLEM IN SOME DEGREE WITH EXCESS FRUCTOSE. This page is a must read if you want to have a successful weight loss program.** *There may be a number of culprits that produce belly fat, but fructose heads the list.* Fructose is found in nature in small amounts in fruits and vegetables and in small amounts it is more beneficial than destructive.

The commercial food industry has produced sweet syrups from corn that is high in fructose. This high fructose corn syrup is hidden in many products you may use frequently without thinking they are that sweet. Products such as ketchup, mustard, seasoning sauces, breakfast bars, your favorite salad dressing, and tempting quick and easy snacks and meal replacement foods can contain high fructose corn syrup. *Why use so much fructose?* Because it is inexpensive and has a long shelf life, from a commercial point of view fructose is an efficient way to sweeten food. This commercial love affair with fructose over the past 70 years, with a huge increase in the past 30 years, has changed the course of disease in this country.

High fructose consumption is a huge problem because it bypasses the digestive system and goes to the liver. The liver says, "I don't like you either." The liver turns it into fat and stores it in the liver or in the belly. **This is the reason for an epidemic increase in belly fat, fatty liver, diabetes and irritable bowel symptoms.**

People trying to lose weight listen up!!! Your brain does not recognize the fructose in high fructose corn sugar or corn syrup as food. Since your body is not nutritionally satisfied, *you do not get the message you are full so you want to eat more.*

Clearly a place to start in weight control is to first eliminate all high fructose foods. They include honey, all tropical fruits like bananas, pineapple, mango, papaya, corn syrup and high fructose corn syrup, and fruit juices that contain more fructose than a single piece of fruit. Also keep in mind that sugarcane is 50% fructose, and agave is 100% fructose. Your best sugar products are Stevia, Coconut Crystals and Coconut Nectar.

For most people low fructose fruits can be eaten one time a day if other health issues are not a concern. These fruits include all berries, all melons, all citrus, peaches, pears, apples, plums, nectarines, cherries, apricots and other local fruit grown in this country. A healthy diet can handle 5-15 grams of fructose daily. Unfortunately, Americans now consume as much as 90 grams of fructose daily that is equivalent to eating 25 peaches in one day. **The natural fructose in low fructose fruit is absorbed slowly … so remember moderation!!!** *Most people should not be afraid to eat fresh organic low fructose fruit one time a day.* Staying clear of the sugary desserts, regular soda drinks and processed food is a good place to start … and **learn to read labels.**

WEIGHT LOSS TIP #15

RESTAURANT FOOD

This clearly depends on whether you are having an occasional celebration like a birthday or anniversary … or you eat out a lot … or are traveling for a week or longer. *The 1ˢᵗ rule is not to order foods you know will make you sick.* During your weight loss effort your **attitude** about how much you deserve to be successful says a lot about your will power. *If you go into a restaurant like a kid in a candy store and then feel deprived if you have to compromise, you need to look at the value you place on yourself.* Except for a few very special occasions, a restaurant meal should just be an extension of the good choices you make every day. *Some guidelines are:*

1. **NEVER** order animal products with hormones and antibiotics unless you have no choice. I never order beef or dairy products, pork, turkey, chicken or eggs. Order ocean fish and only order farm raised fish if there is no other choice. Farm raised fish includes tilapia, catfish, rockfish, bluefish, trout and salmon. Farm raised salmon can also have red food dye added, so always order Pacific or wild salmon and not Atlantic salmon that is farm raised.

2. **NEVER** order anything deep fried as the oil may be rancid since they may only change the oil weekly, or they may just strain it and add more oil. A four star restaurant usually changes the oil daily, but deep fried food is still not recommended because the high heat damages the oil.

3. **NEVER** drink city water from the restaurant. You should be carrying energized water with you so you can drink ½-1 glass before you eat. If you do not have water with you, ask for non-carbonated bottled water. **NEVER** order carbonated water, as that leeches out calcium that you need to balance pH. *Restaurant ice has been tested and can contain bacteria, so ask for an empty glass with no ice and pour in your own healthy water.*

4. **NEVER** drink hot liquids with your meal as it WILL interfere with enzyme activity. So, skip the hot tea. I won't even discuss coffee … OK I will. Coffee dehydrates and over stimulates the pancreas, liver and adrenals that are **TRYING TO DIGEST AND PROCESS YOUR MEAL … THE FOOD THAT KEEPS YOU ALIVE!!!** *Don't mess with Mother Nature.* Most food has good points and bad points, so if you insist on a food that has some bad points then at least remember MODERATION!

5. **NEVER** drink alcohol with your meal as it enlarges the pores of the intestines letting undigested food and toxic wastes go through that **makes your liver mad at you.** Just because some people, even whole countries, take alcohol with their meals does not make it healthy. *Worldwide disease and life expectancy statistics suggest there could be improvement by all countries!!!*

6. **NEVER** eat a sweet dessert that can ferment in the stomach while you are digesting protein. You can take it home to enjoy in a relaxed environment several hours later if it is a special occasion.

THE FOLLOWING RESTAURANT CHOICES MAY BE TOLERATED:

- Buffalo is a red meat that is low in fat and fast becoming popular in restaurants. Do not order buffalo if your saliva pH is below 6.6 because you will not digest it well. Eating hard to digest protein without knowing your saliva pH can be compared to walking into traffic and pretending that a car will not hit you. **We get sick … or overweight … because we are not healthy enough to process the food we eat.**

-   Lamb is another red meat that is easier to digest because the fat is marbled on the outside of the meat and not through the meat like beef and pork. Lamb is generally hormone and antibiotic free. If your saliva pH is at least 6.6, lamb can be helpful to add variety in restaurant choices.

-   Duck is on the menu in most Chinese, Thai and some Mexican restaurants. It is hormone and antibiotic free and can give you delicious choices from the usual selections.

-   Cornish hen and quail should be free of hormones and antibiotics. They are on a lot of menus but most people pass them by for more familiar choices.

-   Ocean fish is preferred, but not farm raised choices unless you have no other options. Many recipes are loaded with ingredients you do not want. Most restaurants will accommodate special requests and simply broil fresh ocean fish for you.

-   Shellfish should be considered over protein that has hormones and antibiotics if there is not a good ocean fish on the menu. Crab is better than shrimp because crab comes from the claw or legs of the crab and does not have the intestinal vein like shrimp. In a good restaurant if you order large shrimp or prawns, the intestinal vein will be removed. I often request a special sauce of olive oil, garlic, lemon juice and real butter that most restaurants will accommodate. I do not go back to any restaurant that will not cooperate with special requests.

- Salad can be individualized by asking what it contains and requesting foods be eliminated that you do not like. I always ask for **NO** head lettuce because of the unwanted chemicals and lower nutritional value. I prefer dark leaf lettuce or spring mix. Salad dressing can be a problem if you have a lot of food concerns. You can always ask for olive oil, vinegar, garlic and lemon. This does not work for travel, but if you are out for a single meal you can bring a small container of your own favorite dressing from home. I tend to stay away from salad bars because people stocking the salad bar may not always wash the vegetables well, and I've seen people reach in for food with their hands.

- Grains can be a problem in a restaurant. If you have a grain allergy you MIGHT do better eating white bread or pasta than whole grains because lower protein means less allergic reaction. You can choose rice noodles over wheat noodles, and you may have fewer problems with wheat and gluten grains if you pick a Mexican, Chinese, Thai or Japanese restaurant. If you should not eat bread always ask them not to bring it because it is tempting sitting on the table.

- Choose rice over potatoes, since commercial potatoes can be treated with multiple chemicals! More restaurants are now serving baked sweet potatoes that may be tolerated by people who cannot eat white potatoes.

You should eat organic at home and order the best you can during your *night out, trip or vacation.* **If you stay in a kitchen unit when you travel you can make an organic breakfast, a shaker drink for lunch and only eat out one time a day.** If you are traveling for a special occasion and choose to order selections you do not usually eat, evaluate how you react. If you get away with little or mild reaction then one meal occasionally is not a problem. *However, if one meal or multiple meals of the wrong selection makes you feel bad, you may decide cheating is not worth the way you feel.*

Be careful if you eat foods you KNOW you should not eat and

do not get sick right away. Thinking you did all right may encourage you to continue choosing wrong foods and one day **YOU FEEL TERRIBLE!!! COLLECTIVE BUILD UP OF SYMPTOMS CAN KNOCK YOU DOWN WHEN YOU LEAST EXPECT IT … AND YOU MIGHT NOT EVEN BLAME THE SLOW CHEATING. Allergic reactions** to food produce symptoms within an hour after eating. **Digestive reactions** to food can take up to several hours. **Chemical reactions** to foods like the nightshades and salicylates can be accumulative over weeks or months. Just like an addictive drug, foods can have an addictive hold on you. **As you crave the food you eat more … and more … and gain weight as your body becomes imbalanced from the abnormal stress. DO NOT FOCUS ON WEIGHT LOSS … FOCUS ON WHAT IS CAUSING YOUR ABNORMAL BODY STRESS. LEARN TO EAT TO LIVE INSTEAD OF LIVING TO EAT!!!**

Enjoy your life … but be reasonable and responsible in your selections!

WEIGHT LOSS TIP #16

POLLUTED FREQUENCIES

Now it is time to get to a serious health problem that robs you of the energy you need for normal body function … including weight control. In the last 50 years we have become a society of polluted frequencies that have changed the world forever. We now live in a world that is dominated by electrical equipment and products, polluted frequencies from computers, power lines, cells phone, beepers, microwaves and oversized TVs, and children obsessed with electronic games. We also live in a world of angry and frustrated people that impact the health of people around them with vibrations from negative emotions. *Your body uses internal energy BORROWED FROM NORMAL BODY FUNCTION to protect you from all polluted, scrambling frequencies. Too often, the exposure exceeds your ability to protect you from these invading frequencies and* **reduces the quality of very important body functions.**

What is stress? One explanation is the opposing reaction of a body resisting a force. That force in modern American is different than any other time in the history of the world. We can no longer maintain the body energy we need for normal body function when we must struggle daily, even hourly to resist so many negative frequencies that are foreign to the body. **Protecting yourself with products that deflect negative frequencies is a must in modern times because IT PROTECTS THE QUALITY OF LIFE AND CAN BE LIFE SAVING.**

Not all technology is bad. Fortunately, good technology has also produced ways to divert negative frequencies away from you. The

BioElectric Shield will deflect all negative frequencies; check www. bioelectricshield.com for information. *One day my BioElectric Shield was being energized in the window at home. I went to a computer store to purchase a faster computer and forgot to wear my shield. The whole store was full of turned on computers and televisions. Without the shield I was shocked how my concentration diminished, my pulse raced, and I felt dizzy and nauseated. I needed to stay and make a decision about the purchase, so I borrowed my husband's shield. In only a few minutes my pulse slowed down, and I felt able to think clearly again.* **That was a dramatic reality check about life with modern technology!**

An additional preventative healthcare tool is Tachyon Technology that is a MUST protection for cell phones, digital cordless phones, computers, television, electronic equipment and games. *This is not a substitute for the BioElectric Shield that has broader protection to all indoor and outdoor negative frequencies.* **You do need extra protection right next to your ear since an unprotected cell phone is like talking with your head in a microwave; cordless phones are potentially even more dangerous.** Do not forget protection for your children and their computer toys. Children are now getting adult diseases. For more information check www.tachyonpartners.com/hmwellness. **Tachyon Technology has many products that help protect our energy for normal body function.**

This health tip is really big!!!!! Your adrenal glands control allergies, mental and emotional stress, chemicals and polluted frequencies. If the stress of living in modern America wipes out your adrenal glands you will not convert thyroid outside the thyroid (discussed in Weight Loss Tip #17) or get the energy value of your food (metabolism). Instead your food is stored as fat. You are beginning to get a picture of *how to survive living in modern America ...**maintain your health and your weight.*** Protect your internal energy from polluted frequencies because everything that goes on in every cell of your body every second of your life is an energy reaction. Exhaust your internal energy and you set the stage for a lot of health problems!

Hope you will soon have an unscrambled day.

WILSON SYNDROME

Most doctors recognize only one way in which the thyroid can fail. If the gland's output of thyroid hormone drops, blood tests will reflect the decrease. But there is another way, one that, while often written about in medical journals is still unknown to most physicians. You could suffer from the effects even if the thyroid gland itself works just fine. In fact, you can have the symptoms associated with the problem even if you are already taking thyroid medication. This second route to thyroid function failure takes place outside of the gland. To have an optimal working of the thyroid gland the body must convert most of the hormone the thyroid secretes (T4) into a five times more active compound called T3. Some people because of continued stress convert T4 into *reverse* T3. Doctor E. Denis Wilson called this Wilson's Syndrome.

Dr. Wilson notes that the condition is one of the body's common responses to stress. That can be anything from starting a new diet, single or multiple pregnancies, major illness or an emotional crisis.

Body temperature is the most reliable way to determine thyroid activity at home. The farther below the normal basal temperature of 98.6F you are, the more likely your thyroid is below par. This temperature should be done first thing in the morning before you move out of bed.

The more symptoms you have, the more probable it is that low thyroid function is the correct diagnosis. Remember while the thyroid tests say that everything is normal your low temperature check still can point to the disorder.

If a person is taking thyroid replacement medication and symptoms persist, something is obviously wrong. As some people continue on either a low calorie or low carbohydrate diet, they often find it increasingly difficult to lose weight. The reason this happens, according to the study, is that the T4 to the T3 conversion diminished while the conversion to reverse T3 (remember that is biologically inert) increased and the body says "where's the thyroid?" This uneven distribution of T3 can create any of the symptoms listed below:

SYMPTOMS COMMONLY CAUSED BY
LOW BODY TEMPERATURE

Fatigue/lethargy	Unhealthy hair
Headaches	Hair loss
Migraines	Insomnia
Irritable Bowel Syndrome	Allergies
Constipation	Hives
Easy weight gain or underweight	Asthma
Decreased memory & concentration	Itchiness
Depression	Dry eyes/Blurred Vision
Fluid retention	Ringing in the ears
PMS/Menstrual Disorders	Abnormal swallowing sensations
Carpal Tunnel Syndrome	Muscle & joint aches
Infertility	Irritability
Anxiety & Panic Disorders	Slow healing
Low motivation & ambition	Bruising easily
Fibromyalgia	Cold hands/Raynaud's phenomenon

Uncontrollable need to sleep	Intolerance to cold/heat
Low sex drive	Flushing/sweating abnormalities
Dry skin & hair	Immune weakness
Acne	Chronic Infection (sinus,bladder,skin)
Brittle nails	Hoarseness

WEIGHT LOSS TIP #18

ENERGY HEALING

BY NOW YOU SHOULD KNOW HEALTH AND WEIGHT CONTROL IS ALL ABOUT ENERGY!!! *Learning how to move your own **ENERGY** for increased health and vitality is the first step to weight control. Any book on physics will tell you that energy cannot be destroyed, but it can travel and leave you weak as it leaves the body.* Energy healing is not designed to diagnose or treat. *If you seek safer, simple, free methods of encouraging your body to heal itself, then working **WITH** nature and not **AGAINST** it may help you achieve the health results ... and weight loss you want.*

"THE FLOW OF ENERGY IS ESSENTIAL TO WELLNESS. DISEASE IS THE RESULT OF ANY INTERFERENCE WITH THIS FLOW."

Ilya Prigogine (Nobel Prize Recipient)

There are 12 main pathways of energy in the body called meridians. The Triple Warmer is the meridian that takes all the bumps, bruises and traumas to protect your body. *Unlike other meridians that relate to major organs, the Triple Warmer does not connect to any specific organ **but guards them all for optimum harmony and balance. The Triple Warmer is the immune system for the meridians. The meridians send energy to all the vital organs.*** The Triple Warmer rests those meridians in case of a catastrophic stress like a poisonous bite, or any emotional or physical shock. *In modern America, we have polluted frequencies from power lines, computers, television, cell phone, beepers, microwaves and* *electronic equipment in our homes, cars and workplace. We are eating, breathing, wearing and sleeping with chemically produced products. We have social, financial and career stresses. Modern drinking water is filtered dead water with no molecular energy, or we drink liquids we think are substitutes for water ... and either drink too much or not enough water. Juice, coffee and sodas have become America's water. Our food is too often nutritionally deficient and full of chemicals and we as a society tend to eat too much food with poor digestion. All the above, plus taking prescription and non-prescription drugs and having both necessary and unnecessary surgeries have become a way of life in modern America for the past 50 years!* **THE TRIPLE WARMER ACTS LIKE IT HAS TO SAVE US EVERYDAY!!!**

When you need your Triple Warmer in case of body shock it will be there for you, but keeping your Triple Warmer calm in day by day living is your first consideration to protect your energy! This is a big part of learning how to survive living in the insane stress of modern America.

The following instructions help you find the points that calm the Triple Warmer and support body energy and balance:

THE FIRST THREE ARE EXTREMELY IMPORTANT:

1. Take 3 fingers of one hand and **firmly** press the opposite temple and **with a continuous firm forward push,** move up over the ear, down behind the ear, halfway down the neck muscle and go over the top of the shoulder. Continue down the arm over the outside elbow bone and firmly push the energy into the 4th finger (next to your little finger). Grab the whole finger and pull the energy out the end of the finger and throw it away. *Do not lift the pressure once you start the push at the temple.* Repeat 3-4 times each arm. **This is the Triple Warmer Meridian** and the routine is best done with no clothes on as you cannot successfully push the energy out of the meridian if you lift your hand going over clothes or jewelry. I do this one time as soon as I get out of bed before I put my robe on and again in the shower at night. **GETTING THE ENERGY OUT**

OF THE TRIPLE WARMER SO YOUR WORKING MERIDIANS CAN BE STRONGER IS YOUR 1ˢᵀ LINE OF DEFENSE IF YOU FEEL WIPED OUT FROM STRESS OR ILLNESS.

2. **Firmly** tap your thymus (the inflammation control part of your immune system) 15-30 seconds at the **top of the breastbone (the bone in the middle of the chest) just below the indentation in your neck** with 4 fingers of either hand. You can tap the thymus **every 30 minutes to 1 hour** if you feel any inflammatory, cold or flu symptoms. You should be able to reduce or prevent these symptoms if you tap your thymus at least four times every day.

3. Put your index fingers of both hands on the boney prominences of your collar bone at **both sides** of the hole in your neck, and the middle and ring finger of each hand placed in the soft tissue under the boney prominence on each side of the breastbone; tap **firmly** with the 3 fingers for 15-30 seconds. This is the 27ᵗʰ place on the kidney meridian that acts like a **whole body stabilizer** ... *think me Tarzan as you tap ... and tap anytime you feel a loss of strength. This master meridian point will give you energy if you tap it at least four times every day.*

THE NEXT FOUR ARE VERY IMPORTANT:

4. Place the thumbs on both sides of the temples just above where the side arms of glasses cross to the ear. Then put 3 fingers on the forehead going straight up from the top of the nose (like you are massaging a headache), and massage **firmly** both the forehead and the temples at the same time 15-30 seconds. This calming action can be done anytime during the day but should be done at least morning and evening.

5. Place the thumb on the palm of the opposite hand for support, wrap your fingers around the little finger side of the

hand, and **firmly** tap or massage the soft tissue **between** the bones of the little finger and ring finger for 15-30 seconds. If you have long fingernails, you can rub sideways in this area. This calms the Triple Warmer and should be done at least two times a day.

6. The brain gets the energy it needs for sharp thinking by the left side of the brain crossing over to energize the right side, and the right side of the brain crossing over to energize the left side of the brain. *When the body is out of balance, the brain does not cross over, causing loss of brain energy.* I'm sure you've heard someone say or thought yourself, "I can't think well today." Encourage your brain to cross over by tapping your right hand to your left knee and crossing over with your left hand to your right knee, 20 taps on each knee. Make sure you cross the arms over to tap the opposite knee, and not just move them sideways. **This will sharpen the brain … every time!** This exercise is very helpful for people who are studying, taking exams, giving speeches, etc. *I know a young boy who was taking an exam and could not remember the answer to a question. Remembering how his mother taught him this exercise, he crossed his arms 20 times under the desk, looked at the question again and answered it correctly.*

7. Tap 15-30 seconds **to the side of each breast** area on the rib cage *½ distance between* the breast nipple and your side straight down from your under arm pit. This routine energizes the spleen, the largest organ of your lymphatic system. *Tap this lymphatic meridian more often along with tapping the thymus area (number 2) if you have any inflammatory symptoms.*

If you want training tapes and books on Energy Healing, contact Donna Eden at 1-800-835-8332 or www.innersource.net. **THIS KNOWLEDGE IS AN EXCITING ADDITION TO YOUR ENERGY HEALING AWARENESS!!!**

PUT BLAME FOR ENERGY LOSS WHERE IT BELONGS

I have a strong sense of spiritual direction to teach people how to help themselves and others in this national health crisis that affects all Americans in some way. I believe our society desperately needs to **take a stand against** our shocking health statistics. ***WHY* is our country out of control on all levels of morals, spiritual connection (this is positively growing), and mental, emotional and physical self-awareness?** You just have to listen to the news or read a newspaper to hear about children and adult crisis situations **EVERYDAY!** The outrageous obsession children and adults have with poor health choices is a national embarrassment. **WE JOKE ABOUT PEOPLE BEING HEALTH CONSCIOUS!** *We are the only country in the world that calls someone interested in healthy choices a health nut.* The typical American lifestyle results in an epidemic of diseases and overweight people who flock to the medical profession for crisis control. **WE ARE A SOCIETY BLINDLY SEARCHING IN THE WRONG PLACES FOR ANSWERS TO INSANE SOCIAL BEHAVIOR.** We teach our children not to run into the street and then feed them refined, chemical junk food that can only make them more unresponsive to other daily teachings. Relationships, careers and social pressures are often being handled by people who themselves have EXHAUSTING chronic health problems. Pacifying the self with unhealthy temptations is easy in a mentally and physically exhausted body. *Here is a list of issues **we need to look at** that influence our energy ... and our choices:*

- **We need to look at** how hard work and goals are interrupted by chronic and acute health issues because people have not learned to pace themselves living the 'American Dream.'

- **We need to look at** how often our *energy level* does not keep up with our hopes and dreams ... **and we spend our lives wishing for what might have been.**

- **We need to look at** our intake of social drugs and addictive habits that influence both the individual and family members.

- **We need to look at** our intake of prescription drugs that are given for chronic symptoms and not just given for acute life saving reasons. *WE NEED TO INSIST ON **WHY THE** AVERAGE PERSON HAS A CHRONIC SYMPTOM INSTEAD OF BLOCKING THE SYMPTOM WITH DRUGS ... NEVER TAKING THE TIME TO FIND THE CAUSE.*

- **We need to look at** the poor quality of many supplements that cannot help. Take supplements that are vegetarian, whole food based and organic.

- **We need to look at** all the exposures to electromagnetic polluted frequencies in our industrialized world that rob us of our energy.

- **We need to look at** the chemical overload we have created in the past 50 years in our food, water, clothing and environment.

- **We need to look at** the changes we have made with too many positive ions and too few negative ions from our modern day environment and cement cities.

- **We need to look at** our children and ask ourselves why they are having adult diseases, and why a leading unit being added to hospitals across this country is the cancer ward for children. **We need to look at** the increase in childhood autism, hyperactivity and other diseases and the connection they may have with infant and preschool vaccinations.

- **We need to look at** kidney dialysis units being added to many hospitals to support kidneys that can no longer handle the insanity of modern America.

- **We need to look at** the decline in family unity. We need more quality family time, relaxing family dinners, and playing old fashion games together. We need to look at the time children spend away from the family in a long list of endless classes and being kept occupied with the latest computer toy and television programs. We think we are educating and helping our children but end up without enough time to sit and play a game or just talk.

There is no humor on this page … this is not funny!

WHAT DOES THIS HAVE TO DO WITH WEIGHT CONTROL? WHAT YOU THINK ABOUT YOURSELF AND YOUR FAMILY UNIT HAS A LOT TO DO WITH THE STRESSORS THAT AFFECT YOUR CHOICES!!!

WEIGHT LOSS TIP #19

STRESS MANAGEMENT

Stress is a killer ... setting a person up to make bad choices that adds to the stress ... and contributes to chronic and acute symptoms as well as weight gain. **We can't avoid being stressed, but we can control the damage from the stress response with four main minerals.** *Sodium and calcium turn on the stress response, and magnesium and potassium turn off the stress response.* **When these minerals are OUT OF BALANCE, stress gets out of control.** In 1840, a German scientist named Justus Von Liebig discovered that when only nitrogen, potassium and phosphorus were put back into the soil, farmers could grow crops on the same piece of land over and over again without rotating crops. *Liebig is the father of artificial fertilizer that skyrocketed productivity and profit.* **The plants looked healthy because they could survive with just the three minerals and water, but people who ate those plants became mineral deficient.** If *WE* want to be healthy, we have to give the plants *ALL THE MINERALS WE NEED, NOT JUST THE ONES THE PLANTS NEED.* Commercial food can be magnesium deficient. Without magnesium you cannot turn off the stress response, so people struggle with poor stress management. **ORGANIC FOOD IS THE HEALTH FOOD OF THE FUTURE!!!**

Your nervous system has two main controls ... one for normal stress days and one for emergency stress situations. During a crisis, energy from any body system that is not involved in *immediate* survival is sacrificed. That borrowed energy can now go where it is most needed to fight harder during the crisis. *Any acute **traumatic** situation, such*

78

as mental (thinking), emotional (feeling) or physical, is all treated the same as someone being attacked by a wild animal. Modern day stress is an **OVERLOADED** combination of polluted frequencies, chemicals, nutritionally deficient food, social and financial demands, acute and chronic ill health, prescription and non-prescription drugs, and pressure to live the American dream. *This can all cause poor digestion, weaken the immune system, turn off the growth and repair systems, impair sleep, obstruct circulatory function and hinder the production of hormones that help us deal with more stress.* **This OVERLOADED collection of stress situations can be seen in ways from chronic symptoms ... to disease ... to weight gain. Long term stress makes it difficult, if not impossible, for the body to keep up with the normal needs required for healthy body functions.**

Cortisol is one of many hormones secreted by your adrenal glands in response to any type of stress. *Its levels are normally highest in the morning to wake you up and lowest at night to let you sleep.* If your levels are low in the morning you will have a hard time waking up and could feel tired all day. If your levels are high at night you could be depressed and have trouble sleeping. Your cortisol levels respond to daily stress but should re-adjust after each event. **When your adrenals keep secreting this hormone inappropriately from constant stress, it can exhaust the adrenal glands ... and leave you feeling sick and tired of being sick and tired!!!** Besides that, excess cortisol pulls calcium out of your bones, puts you at risk for losing bone density and can be stored in abdominal tissue causing that middle bulge. You can regulate cortisol levels naturally with the **laws of wellness** and whole food B complex supplements. The classification of supplement herbs called adaptogens regulates your body's response to stress. Some herbs are nutritional, some are cleansing and some are adaptogens specific for stress management. Look for the word 'adaptogens' when shopping for herbal formulas to help you deal with the stressors of living in modern America. The Russians first discovered the value of adaptogen herbs that made them outstanding in space travel, Olympics and aging.

All higher brain functions become suppressed in stress, so you can concentrate on the fight or flight emergency needs. We actually have three brains. The **reptile brain** is in charge of reflexes and survival and is **90-100% selfish**. *All selfish negative emotions energize the reptile brain.* When people are being controlled by that part of their brain, you cannot expect much cooperation out of them for your problems because they are processing from a selfish point of view. The best thing you can do is wait for things to pass, as moods always change. The **mammal brain** gives us emotions, social skills and is **50% or more cooperative, capable of some acts of self-sacrifice**. *The mammal brain is the center for emotions, both positive and negative, but the negative does not come from selfish thoughts.* The **human brain** gives us language, reasoning and creativity. *We have large, powerful, creative and sensitive prefrontal lobes, and we are capable of greater acts of love, creativity, unselfishness and cooperation than the rest of the creatures on this earth.* **Stress suppresses everything except the reptile brain, which beats the heart and moves the lungs.** *In a crisis situation you cannot be as nice a person (mammal brain suppressed) or as smart or creative (human brain suppressed).*

SO HOW DO YOU HELP A BAD MOOD PASS AND ACTIVATE YOUR MAMMAL OR HUMAN BRAIN:

1. Appreciation for someone else is an unselfish act.

2. Even in a bad day you can thank God for the lessons to be learned, and consciously look for the positive elements of the day.

3. Focus on your feelings rather than your reactions.

4. Distract yourself from the stressful thoughts by getting involved in something that interests you. When your mood lifts (and it will), rethink the problem and your creative brain will come up with an idea.

All the collective information you learn will help you deal with the stress of living in modern America. **The one result I consistently get from my wellness program is my clients admitting that they are**

calmer and able to deal with stress better. There is not one single recommendation … **all the laws of wellness** need to be understood in order to survive the challenges of recent decades. *Think of all the millions of people in America who do not understand what is happening to them.*

YOU ARE THE LUCKY ONE!!!

WEIGHT LOSS TIP # 20

NATURAL FOOD SUPPLEMENTS

In this world of multiple stress issues, your supplement program is more important than ever before. Providing a healthy nutritional base for normal body function starts your wellness effort needed for weight control. If you went to a health food store and looked at the rows of supplements, *OR* read all the supplement advertising in your frequently stuffed mailbox, *OR* talked to your friends who may not pass along accurate advice, you are thoroughly confused about supplementation. Even worse, if you shop for supplements at a grocery store, discount or chain store, you are most likely getting products that are incompatible with **YOUR CHEMISTRY ...** but very compatible with the supplement company's and the store owner's profits. *Every company tries to convince you their products can pull off the fountain of youth promise.* Even doctor's offices carry what you assume are good supplements because ... *a doctor recommended them.* **Unfortunately, commercial and profit seeking companies are interested in ... guess what ... profit!!!** In the Spring 2006 Health & Healing Consumer Alert newsletter by Julian Whitaker, M.D., it states, *"Is alternative medicine selling out? Natural healing has achieved so much and we've never needed it more. But is this lifesaving crusade turning into a cynical gold rush? Hordes of hucksters are swarming in, peddling unproven 'cures' that cost hundreds or thousands of dollars per month ..."* Robert Rowen M.D., in his Consumer's Heart Health News (available 1-800-728-2288) Winter Issue 2006 states, *"In independent lab test 57% of the policosanol brands (for cholesterol) tested FAILED to meet basic standards. Some contained as little as 23% of the amount of policosanol listed on the label! It's bad* *enough these sleazy supplement makers are cutting costs by cheating on their potencies. But they're also using cheap substitutes to pump up their profits. And they're skimping on one crucial ingredient that's essential to getting the results you want."* Since biofeedback equipment to verify the compatibility of a product with **your** chemistry is not yet in most doctors' offices, recommendations are too often a **GUESSING GAME BASED ON A SALES PITCH OR PRINTED ADVERTISING, AND NOT ON YOU AS A BIOCHEMICAL INDIVIDUAL!!!**

Food is the primary factor in nutrient delivery and utilization. *Many commercial supplements are made in a chemist's lab and are look-a-likes to a fraction of a whole complex. In that form they are treated in the body like a drug, and not as a physiologically supporting nutrient like supplements derived from food sources.* Because of the intense competition among so many supplement companies, *price has become the most important feature of their product line ...* **and lower prices too often can mean lower quality!!!** Supplements derived from food sources cost more to manufacture, so commercial profit seekers have hopped on the 'money train' given the current health trends, and are more interested in your purchase than the value you receive. ***Considering the number of people buying supplements, our health statistics should be better.*** You can buy a book on kinesiology muscle testing and learn how to test your energy compatibility with the energy of the supplement. *If the supplement is good for you, your arm will be very strong ... and if you are weakened by the energy of the supplement you will feel weak on the arm testing.* Learn to muscle test before you base your health on any supplement recommendation or personal guessing game.

In my opinion, the following supplements are worth considering:

1. *For over 30 years* **MEGAFOOD** *has been a leader in providing pure, bio-available and effective food nutrients. MegaFood was the first company in 1973 to recognize the importance of natural food sources in the delivery of nutrients.* **Their supplements are organic, vegetarian,**

soy free, 100% whole food or herbal derived, and highly absorbed. They have a number of nutritional supplements from this company that are generally safer for anyone with specific health concerns. **Any company that goes to the expense of making it vegetarian will be more conscious of other quality control factors. MegaFood is a company I recommend without hesitation because they use full color spectrum food-based nutrition that is the next best thing to eating whole food, and they are available in most health food stores or health pharmacies.** You can check out their whole line at www.megafood.com.

2. **ROYAL BODY CARE** *is a multi-level company* that requires a distributor number to order. You can use mine (10984) because I am **not interested in building a business, and you will never get called or pressured by me to buy more than you want or to be a distributor.** They sell organic Spirulina that is extremely well absorbed for anyone dealing with the stress of living in modern America. Spirulina is one of the few foods on earth you can live on with just it and water. *I consider Royal Body Care a higher quality source for Spirulina than wild grown Spirulina.* The contact number is 1-800-722-0444.

3. **SPROUTED FLAXSEED** is better absorbed than any other version of flaxseed. It is a super food and provides essential fats, vitamins, minerals and enzymes. Whole seeds are difficult to digest so the body does not get all the nutritional value of flax. When flax seed is milled it improves digestibility, but it can turn rancid if not used up in about a month. No other form of flax is as stable and can compare to the nutritional availability of *ORGANIC SPROUTED FLAXSEED.*

4. **MACA ROOT** has been used by the Peruvian Indians back to 3800 B.C. for nutritional and medicinal value. *Maca contains amino acids, carbohydrates, vitamins and minerals,*

has a tonic effect on the whole body, enhances all glandular function, regulates hormones, and is an adaptogen that helps your body defend itself against physical and mental stress. Maca comes in capsules as well as loose powder and is available in most health food stores.

5.   **VITAMIN D3** may be an important supplement addition because many people spend little time outdoors year round, and people who do love being in the sun are obsessed with using commercial sun blockers. I read an article that states many babies are born with a Vitamin D deficiency because of not enough sun or too much sun blockers used by the mother. Make sure you are getting Vitamin D3 (cholecalciferol) and not D2 (ergocalciferol) found in synthetic vitamins. If you feel pain pressing firmly on your sternum (breastbone) you may be suffering from Vitamin D deficiency. Vitamin D may be the single most underrated nutrient involved in many health concerns like calcium absorption that controls pH. The dose during the winter months (or even year round if you are mostly an indoor person) is an average of 3000-4000 mg daily. Always look for vegetarian supplements.

6.   **EMU OIL HEALS!** The emu bird is a native to Australia and has fast become a success story for many producers in this country. **Emu oil is one of nature's best kept secrets.** The *outstanding results* using the oil both as an internal supplement and a skin product have made a *huge demand* for many emu products now being produced. Emu oil is made up of essential fatty acids and is the oil that is most like the oil our bodies produce. Every day our bodies are producing 300 billion new cells, and each cell needs essential fatty acids to build a strong cell wall. Emu oil starts repairing and nourishing new cells … *a good place to start building your new healthier and thinner body. It is fast becoming a favorite among skincare and health care professionals… one source is* www.ThunderRidgeEmu.com

*SUPPLEMENT CHOICES SHOULD ALWAYS REFLECT A BOND WITH NATURE. In nature and in the body, vitamins are found in combination with other factors. An extracted vitamin may be structurally identical to a part of the whole, but the functional role of the whole form will act differently in connection with other factors. It should also be noted that there is a danger in taking too many supplements that contain all the trace minerals. **Remember, they are called trace minerals, not unlimited minerals!** Too much of a good thing does not make it better.* **YOUR SUPPLEMENT CHOICES SHOULD PROVIDE AN EXTENSION OF HEALTHY FOODS. INSTEAD OF CAUSING MORE IMBALANCE, SUPPLEMENTS SHOULD ASSIST IN YOUR EFFORT TO BALANCE YOUR CHEMISTRY.**

HOMEOPATHY

IF YOU HAVE A SYMPTOM FROM HEADACHE TO WEIGHT GAIN, YOUR VITAL FORCE IS DOWN! IT IS YOUR DEPRESSED VITAL FORCE, NOT YOUR SYMPTOMS OR WEIGHT GAIN THAT IS YOUR PROBLEM. Homeopathy is a method of stimulating the body's own healing process in order to allow the body to heal itself. The word homeopathy is taken from the Greek homeos meaning similar and pathos meaning suffering. Thus, homeopathy means to treat with something that produces an effect similar to suffering. *IT IS THE LAW OF SIMILARS … OR … LIKE CURES LIKE.*

Homeopathy holds that every person has a vital or dynamic force, which normally keeps the person healthy by maintaining a *normal balance of all systems* in the body, mind and spirit. Homeopathy thus defines **all disease** whether physical, mental or emotional, acute or chronic … **as derangements of the vital force in an attempt to restore balance.** This derangement occurs at such a subtle level that it cannot be directly perceived except through '**symptoms.**' *All symptoms are created by the vital force in its struggle to maintain balance and health.* **Homeopathic medicine views all symptoms however painful or disagreeable as beneficial, in that they point out the *path* that the vital force has taken in its attempt to restore health.**

Homeopathy works on the principle of RESONANCE … like a singer who shatters glass on a special note that **MATCHES** the energy of the glass. The source of the homeopathic remedy can be *any substance* that has *proven* to have certain symptoms when taken in excess. When the *proven* symptoms **EXACTLY MATCH** the symptoms of the person, the **TWO** energies **combined** will increase the overall energy (called resonance). **This increased energy raises your vital force and you are now stronger to overcome the symptoms.** *The importance in homeopathy is to match LIKE SYMPTOMS ON ALL LEVELS OF PHYSICAL, EMOTIONAL AND MENTAL.* The closer the match of like symptoms on all levels produces the best resonance. You will have no effect from the wrong remedy because there will be no resonance (like a singer who does not break glass). **To change the LEVEL OF HEALTH, change the person's constitution or VITAL FORCE …** *a subtle governing energy that organizes and directs physical and chemical action of the body.* The efficiency of a person's vital force is reflected in degrees of health or illness. *Visualize your vital force between two poles … the lower pole represents as sick as you can get based on your current total health and hereditary factors … and the higher pole represents as healthy as you can get based on your total health and hereditary factors.*

REMEMBER… SYMPTOMS ARE AN EXPRESSION OF YOUR VITAL FORCE'S EFFORT TO HEAL. DO NOT SUPPRESS YOUR BODY'S ATTEMPT TO COMMUNICATE WITH YOU … TUNE INTO BODY LANGUAGE!!! BEING OVERWEIGHT IS NOT JUST A REFLECTION OF EATING TOO MUCH … SO JUST CUTTING DOWN ON FOOD IS NOT ENOUGH TO HEAL THE BODY. Drugs that suppress symptoms should be avoided if possible and only used in acute situations. *Just treating symptoms is masking the fact that your vital force is down and you need to be dealing with that fact rather than just temporarily wanting to feel better or lose weight.* In an acute crisis the traditional approach is comforting, and can be life saving. After the crisis we must always look for the **cause** of the body not working at optimum performance and how to assist the body in healing itself.

You can now collect fast acting and effective homeopathic remedies that will be your first aid kit ready to be **your 1st line of defense.** In many early symptoms homeopathy can raise your vital force to encourage a healing process faster than anything else. There are *tips* to using these remedies, and I suggest you invest in some *beginning homeopathic books.* **This approach to unwanted health changes is not intended to treat or replace appropriate health professionals or medical advice.** *Homeopathy can often keep a simple symptom from becoming a crisis that requires more professional attention.* In homeopathy it is the symptom that guides the remedy choice, while knowing the name of the disease is not necessary. *Homeopathy can be used for almost any symptom. Although serious illnesses should also be monitored by your health care professional, homeopathy can be a fantastic complement to any effort to regain wellness.*

You may find these sources helpful in your homeopathic educational process:

- **Homeopathic Healing Miracles** is a monthly, publication that is a perfect place to start understanding homeopathy, how to care for homeopathic remedies, and important remedies to have on hand for common emergencies. To order an annual subscription call 1-905-760-9929 ext. 300.

- **Washington Homeopathic Products** has a catalog for purchasing remedies. Call 1-800-336-1695 or www. homeopathyworks.com.

- **Standard Homeopathic Co.** has a catalog for purchasing remedies, 1-800-624-9659, or www.hylands.com.

- **Homeopathic Educational Services has a catalog, books, courses, tapes, software, charts (an excellent one-stop source)** 1-800-359-9051 or www.homeopathic.com.

- **Find a local homeopathic healer** who is certified, knowledgeable, patient, and caring. Your health is important, and that caring practitioner holds your health in his/her hands, so make sure you find the most qualified. *These sources may help you find the best in your area:*

    * **The owner or manager of a health food store may know about local homeopathy groups,**

Naturopathic Doctors, or holistic Medical Doctors in the area.

* Pharmacies that carry homeopathic medicines may know local practitioners.

* Alternative magazines and newspapers are often available at health food stores. You are very lucky if you find a Medical Doctor or Naturopathic Doctor who practices homeopathy! Raising your vital force is the best way to produce the health improvement … and weight loss you seek.

WEIGHT LOSS TIP #22

BACH FLOWER REMEDIES

The human body functions using energy on **all levels** of mental, emotional and physical. The Bach Flower Remedies are in the same category as other subtle methods of healing such as homeopathy or herbal medicine. Edward Bach was a highly successful bacteriologist and homeopathic physician, who gave up his lucrative medical practice in 1930 to search for a simpler, more natural method of treatment that did not require anything to be destroyed or altered.

Every physical, emotional or mental symptom gives us a particular message, and we need to acknowledge these messages because *THEY INFLUENCE OUR CHOICES.* **EVERY TRUE HEALING PROCESS IS AN AFFIRMATION OF OUR WHOLENESS.** The Bach Flower remedy system heals by restoring harmony in **AWARENESS.** When vital energies are channeled the wrong way or blocked with negative thoughts, the Bach Flower Remedies re-establish positive contact with our wholeness.

Bach Flower Remedies are different from other subtle methods of treatment in 3 ways:

1. They deal more with ***disharmony in the soul*** in a different way than homeopathic remedies deal with mental and emotional symptoms.

2. The healing energies are released from the flowers in a way that there can be no overdose, no side-effects and no

91

incompatibility with other methods of treatment. The plant itself is not destroyed or damaged. The flower containing all the essential energies of the plant is picked at full perfection when it is about to drop.

3. You do not need to be trained in medicine or psychology to use Bach Flower Remedies. **You only need the *ability to think and acknowledge sensitivities and feelings.***

In 1943 Bach wrote the following incredible insight about his Flower Remedies:

"The action of these remedies is to raise our vibrations and open up our channels for the reception of the Spiritual Self; to flood our natures with the particular virtue we need, and wash out from us the fault that is causing the harm. They are able, like beautiful music or any glorious uplifting thing which gives us inspiration, to raise our very natures, and bring us nearer to our souls and by that very act to bring us peace and relieve our sufferings. They cure, not by attacking the disease, but by flooding our bodies with the beautiful vibrations of our Higher Nature, in the presence of which, disease melts away as snow in the sunshine. There is not true healing unless there is a change in outlook, peace of mind, and inner happiness. Let not the simplicity of this method deter you from its use, for you will find the further your researches advance the greater you will realize the simplicity of all Creation. They who will obtain the greatest benefit from this God-sent Gift will be those who keep it pure as it is; free from science, free from theories, for everything in Nature is simple."

Bach felt that the true causes of disease are the 'defects' from our negative side such as pride, cruelty, hatred, self-love, ignorance, greed, fear, jealousy, anger and worry. He said that two basic errors are the cause of disease:

1. When the personality turns away from love, positive character traits are distorted and become destructive leading to negative moods.

2. The personality turns against the principle of unity and renders the sufferer a slave to his own body.

IF THIS DOES NOT SOUND PROBABLE, THEN UNDERSTAND AND ACCEPT THAT BACH FLOWER REMEDIES HEAL IN A WAY THAT FIRST DOES NO HARM. *Simplicity tends to be misunderstood in a world of increasing sophistication.* Simplicity has to do with unity, perfection and harmony. That is the reason everybody feels attracted to the *'simple things in life.'* The specific flower energy has the same wavelength as the energy of the Higher Self (*your subconscious mind*) wanting to express itself. The remedies are able to connect with your subconscious and change a lower **disharmonious** level to a higher **harmonious** frequency. This new reinforcement is now able to see things in a different light. **This is critical, since disharmony from negative mental and emotional thoughts is a sure way to sabotage weight control.**

BACH FLOWER REMEDIES HELP YOU FIND YOUR TRIPLE P'S …

POSITIVE PERSONAL POWER!!!

The three things that control digestion are positive thinking, water and pH balance. DIGESTION CONTROLS YOUR HEALTH!!! NEVER FORGET THAT IN ANY DISEASE… INCLUDING WEIGHT CHANGES … THERE ARE ONLY THREE BASIC PROBLEMS:

- **NUTRITIONAL STARVATION**

- **TOXIC OVERLOAD**

- **WEAK VITAL FORCE OR CONSTITUTIONAL ABILITY TO STAY HEALTHY**

**** YOUR THOUGHTS CONTROL ALL THREE!!!

Changing the subconscious mind needs as much positive repetition as you gave negative thoughts before. Most health food stores and homeopathic sources carry Bach Flower Remedies that assist in changing from negative to positive thoughts and feelings through **repetitious positive affirmations**. The different Bach Flower Remedies listed here state the negative feelings first, followed by a suggested positive affirmation; or you may choose your own words. *You must state a positive affirmation each time before and after you take the remedy.* **Do you recognize yourself in any of the following?**

AGRIMONY - Attempts to conceal disturbing thoughts behind a façade of cheerfulness.

> *"I am finding peace within myself."*

ASPEN - Apprehensions, fear of some impending evil.

> *"I feel confident and strong."*

BEECH - Arrogance, intolerance, criticizing without understanding the views of others.

> *"I am making peace with myself and others."*

CENTUARY - Weak-willed, easily exploited, can't say no.

> *"I stand up for my own needs."*

CERATO - Doubting own judgment, and having to seek the confirmation of others.

> *"Only I can decide what is right for me."*

CHERRY PLUM - Fear of letting go, fear of losing control, uncontrollable bursts of anger. This remedy is a part of Rescue Remedy.

> *"I accept my calm inner guidance."*

CHESTNUT BUD - Repeating the same faults over and over due to lack of learning from experiences.

> *"I am learning something from every experience."*

CHICORY - Possessive, interfering, manipulating the affairs of others, self-pity, demanding full support from others.

"I respect the boundaries of every individual."

CLEMATIS - Daydreaming, paying little attention to what is going on around you. This remedy is part of Rescue Remedy.

"I am attentive to what is happening now."

CRAB APPLE - Feeling of being unclean, infected, inner disgust with self.

"I am at peace with my mind and body."

ELM - Overwhelmed by responsibility.

"I do the best I can at any given time."

GENTIAN - Skeptical, pessimistic, easily discouraged.

"Obstacles are opportunities to learn."

GORSE - Long term suffering from chronic disease that produces negative expectations and reinforces disease.

"Hope brings healing energy."

HEATHER - Needs an audience to express everything that happens in detail.

"I am secure within myself."

HOLLY - Hatred, envy, jealousy, suspicion.

"I concentrate on my own personal development."

HONEYSUCKLE - Clings to the past, overly nostalgic or homesick.

"I release the past and make myself available in the present."

HORNBEAM - Weariness and exhaustion is largely in the mind.

"I feel awake and refreshed."

IMPATIENS - Impatient, intolerant, irritable. This remedy is part of Rescue Remedy.

"Each part of my journey has its own speed."

LARCH - Lack of self-confidence and fear of failure.

"I can do it; I will do it; I am doing it."

MIMULUS - Shy, timid, fearful.

"My inner strength and courage releases my fear.

MUSTARD - Dark cloud feeling that saddens for no known reason, or powerless feeling.

"My heart feels light and hopeful

OAK - Never knowing when to let go of the fight against great odds.

"I know when it is time to move on in my life journey."

OLIVE - Exhaustion, drained energy on the physical level.

"I feel energy flowing into me."

PINE - Guilt complex blaming self even for the mistakes of others.

"I forgive and love myself."

RED CHESTNUT - Excessive concern and worry over others.

"I radiate optimism and allow others to live their journey."

ROCK WATER - Life's pleasures are suffocated under self-imposed disciplines.

"I am open to new insights and experiences."

ROCK ROSE - Acute state of fear, terror, and panic. This remedy is part of Rescue Remedy.

"I am in God's hands.

SCLERANTHUS - Indecisive, erratic, fluctuating moods.

"The definite decision is within me."

STAR OF BETHLEHEM - Paralyzing sorrow following shocking events. This remedy is part of Rescue Remedy.

"My whole system is calmly breathing."

SWEET CHESTNUT - Hopeless despair; reached the limit of endurance.

"Night has to come before it can be day again."

VERVAIN - Overly enthusiastic, even fanatical.

"I control my energy and learn from others."

VINE - Dominating, inflexible, striving for power.

"I learn from the uniqueness of every individual."

WALNUT - Difficulties adjusting to transition periods of life.

"I dismiss limiting factors that inhibit my journey."

WATER VIOLET - Loners who need to be alone with little emotional involvement.

"I need the world and the world needs me."

WHITE CHESTNUT - Unwanted thoughts keep going around in one's head.

"The solutions I need will come to mind."

WILD OAT - Dissatisfaction with one's mission in life.

"I allow my life journey to guide me in my growth."

WILD ROSE - Resignation, lack of ambition, apathy.

"Life is getting more interesting and beautiful."

WILLOW - Unspoken resentment, bitterness, and victim attitude.

"I am thinking, doing, and achieving positive things."

RESCUE REMEDY - Trauma, numbness, terror, panic, irritability, tension, and fear.

"The calmness deep within me gives me strength and courage."

Bach Flower Remedies do not change the situation. They change your interpretation of the situation. Your new positive interpretations can help you do things differently … make better choices … *and that can change the situation.* WHEN YOU CHANGE YOUR SUBCONSCIOUS TO MORE POSITIVE THINKING, YOU ARE MORE LIKELY TO LOSE THE WEIGHT … AND KEEP THE WEIGHT OFF.

NEVER FORGET THAT YOUR GOAL IS NOT JUST TO LOSE WEIGHT. YOUR GOAL SHOULD ALWAYS BE TO FIND THAT PLACE DEEP INSIDE YOU THAT SAYS YOU ARE AT PEACE WITH THE WORLD … AND WITH YOURSELF. IF YOU DOUBT THAT CAN HAPPEN THEN LISTEN TO THE WORDS YOU SAY TO YOURSELF. CHANGE YOUR NEGATIVE THOUGHTS TO POSITIVE … AND MIRACLES HAPPEN!

I AM BECOMING …

ONLY YOU CAN CHANGE YOUR FUTURE. YESTERDAY IS OVER, TOMORROW HAS NOT COME, BUT OH THE POWER OF TODAY!!!

WEIGHT LOSS TIP #23

GRIEVING PROCESS

The grieving process is a process of growing. Keep in mind that we grieve about many things besides the death of a loved one. We grieve about loss of a relationship, separation and divorce, loss of income or job, loss of goals, moving, retirement, aging, loss of health or youth, loss of beauty or hair, loss from a robbery or fire, loss of control in a situation, loss of hope or pride or self-worth, and loss of your youthful figure. You can have potential losses like a person missing. *Under the burden of each sorrow we either grow … or we die a little each time.* The suffering can give us new strength … or it drains us and robs us of life. The Irish have a saying **"THE SAME FIRE THAT MELTS THE WAX HARDENS THE STEEL."**

Regardless of the reason for the grief, what happens is the most profound pain we'll ever experience. It can strike suddenly and cause havoc for months, years or a lifetime. It can stress our immune system and leave us vulnerable to disease. It can cause virtually every illness from acne to arthritis, headache to heart disease, cold sores to cancer … and weight gain. **ALL BODY SYMPTOMS ARE INFLUENCED FOR BETTER OR WORSE BY OUR EMOTIONS.**

Loss is part of our lives from our beginning when we suffer the loss of protection in our mother's womb … or weaning from breast feeding … or starting school and leaving a familiar routine. Some grieving is easier because it is final and opens up new experiences that help us grow, as time allows healing to occur. Some grieving is bearing a lifetime of unending suffering. *You can get stuck in any one of the first four stages of grieving*

…Denial … Anger … Bargaining … Depression … and never proceed to … Acceptance … that allows you to go on with your life.

"THERE IS NO SUCH THING AS A PROBLEM WITHOUT A GIFT FOR YOU IN HAND."

Richard Bach, Author of "ILLUSIONS"

Some people are **natural survivors** and come through horrible challenges, becoming somehow enriched and renewed. *They all have things in common like choosing not to be a victim, using life's lessons as ways to become stronger, more into 'we' than 'I', and concentrating on their contribution to mankind.*

The **casualties** who physically and emotionally collapse also have things in common. *They hold on to anguish and despair because their belief system is they can't be happy and life is hard, they live in the past and have little energy for the present or future, they build memorials to their losses that give them excuses for their behavior and they create a negative subconscious that traps them.* **Are you still grieving about something?** *There is this example:*

> *Two celibate monks walking near a stream came across a young woman wanting to cross it. One of the monks, to the dismay of the other, picked up the woman and carried her across the stream. About a mile later, the monk who was aghast at the other's action asked how he could pick up a woman when they were supposed to be celibate. The monk replied that he had put the woman down a mile back; why was the other still carrying her around?*

In any loss be gentle with yourself. You have had an emotional wound … but wounds can heal. **There are 3 primary needs for appropriate grief work:**

- **ACKNOWLEDGE THAT YOU HAVE A COMMITMENT TO HEAL** – You cannot go forward by going backwards.

- **ACKNOWLEDGE YOUR SPIRITUAL THERMOSTAT THAT BALANCES EMOTIONS** – You can call your powerful emotional strength anything you want … but it is there when you need it.

- **UNDERSTAND THAT ENERGY IS OUR INWARD NATURE** – Find a way to experience again that feeling of 'getting it all together' that most people have enjoyed at some time during their lives. *The redirection of positive energy is the first step through the grief process.*

The grieving person is mentally weary. An *exhausted* mind distorts reality … that makes it easier to think negative thoughts. *Our physical bodies, emotions and mind are intimately interacting. To ignore the needs of one will sabotage them all … in time.* When emotional pain hurts, you need to take very good care of yourself and make healthy choices for your well-being. A nutritionally deficient system becomes too sensitive, and you react emotionally rather than think a situation through. **GRIEVING IS NOT TIME FOR JUNK FOOD!!!** *Caffeine and alcohol increase urination and deplete needed nutrients. Sodas rob you of calcium at a time when you need three times more calcium than when you are not in stress. This is a time when exercise is critical to get rid of the toxins produced by stress. This is a time to eat organic food and not add chemicals to the burden your system is already experiencing.*

I used to teach a grieving class, and some of my material came from a class I took on grief management. The instructor's story is an example of growing through expressive grief work, having survived her husband's suicide, and four years later her talented son's suicide. She says beautifully:

"We have our bodies with all our marvelous sensory gifts – movement, sound, and vision. We have our intelligence to make plans, study and seek outside help. We have our emotions – everything from apathy, desolation, alienation, to excitement, discovery and intimacy to use. We are equipped to live, learn and mature. If we choose to break loose our stagnant energy, to become active rather than passive, to hope rather than abuse fate, then

by measure we have passed one of the critical tests fulfilling our potential. The choice is mine … and yours."

IF YOU ALLOW YOURSELF TO BECOME STRONGER FROM THE LOSS OR EXPERIENCE, THEN IT GIVES SOME REASON AND VALUE TO THE PAIN YOU ARE FEELING. IT HELPS TO ANSWER THE QUESTION … WHY? IT GIVES PURPOSE TO THAT PART OF LIFE WE DO NOT UNDERSTAND. IT HELPS RENEW YOUR ENERGY! IT HELPS YOU MAKE BETTER CHOICES.

Those better choices that provide energy can start with how you look to yourself and others. The need for energy is plainly seen and felt by the way we dress. Some people make a statement of individuality, others of success and others of innocence. **OUR SELECTION OF COLORS IN ALL AREAS OF OUR LIVES CAN ENERGIZE OUR ACCEPTANCE OR REJECTION OF OURSELVES THROUGH THE ENERGY OF COLOR!**

"Color" refers to a mental and emotional interpretation of what the eyes see. Since sunlight sustains life and there is death without it, man has believed in the healing power of color since the beginning of recorded time. Color was associated with disease because disease produced color – red, inflammation; blue, cold; pale to white for illness; black, blue, yellow, green for degrees of injury. Light and color are being worked back into modern medicine such as infrared radiation for certain aches and pains, ultraviolet light for depression and blue light to treat newborn jaundice.

Color is a vital part of life force **ALL AROUND US!** The use of color in our bodies introduces a natural ENERGY that promotes the elimination of waste products that helps repair cellular damage and encourages positive thinking and enthusiasm. *White is a combination of colors associated with pure, clean and cool. Black is the absence of color associated with neutrality and emptiness.* It is interesting that black has become the basic color in our stressful world. **Health is best achieved using the many shades of visible color that have a powerful influence on our health.** The two extremes of the color spectrum are:

- **RED** raises vital signs and excites body responses. **The hot or advancing colors are red, orange, and yellow.**

- **BLUE** lowers vital signs and relaxes body responses. **The cold or receding colors are turquoise, blue and purple.**

- **GREEN is a neutral color**

The following are ways color influences us:
- **THE FOOD WE EAT** - People who like very few bright colored vegetables and eat mostly meat, dairy, grains and starches are missing an important energy factor that promotes a healthy mind and body. Look at a plate of sliced meat, potatoes and gravy … then add a spread of ripe red tomatoes and notice the difference in your interest. Stir-fry some rice and leftover chicken … then notice the difference when you add tomatoes, green and yellow squash, and red or green peppers to the stir-fry. *Vitamins were discovered by the color present in them.*

- **THE COLORS IN OUR ENVIRONMENT** – If a person's surroundings are bright, that energy will be carried into daily living decisions. Warm colors are best in the kitchen, dining room, recreation and work areas. Cool colors are relaxing and best in the bedroom, sitting room, library or den. Finding a place of peace and quiet by the blue sea or in a green forest could create more spring fever than creativity unless being calm inspires you. **Colors do send signals.** *Have you ever seen a blue stop sign, a turquoise danger sign or a green hazardous area sign?*

- **THE COLORS WE WEAR** – It helps to know what colors look best on your skin tone. Find out if your skin tone is a Spring, Summer, Fall or Winter by being professionally color draped or reading a book on personal colors. It will save you money not buying as many clothes on impulse that once you get them home you do not understand why they just hang in the closet. **The way you dress is a 'color energy' expression of where you are coming from!!!**

I worked in a teenage ward of a psychiatric hospital and one day the parents of a female patient were visiting her. They wanted to go out and buy her some clothes, and she gave them detailed instructions of what she wanted. They returned with a pair of black jeans, black socks, a black top and black sweatshirt. She took the clothes to her room with no change in her expression.

People are born to win...but they must first develop a good self image. Have more to look at when you open your closet than ... is it clean, or is it pressed? **BE DYNAMIC ... DRESS TO WIN AND TURN YOURSELF ON!!! YOUR DRESS SIZE IS NOT AS IMPORTANT AS FEELING ENERGY FROM WHAT YOU WEAR!!!**

WEIGHT LOSS TIP #24

IMMUNE SYSTEM

STAYING A HEALTHY AND NORMAL WEIGHT IS EASY IF YOU UNDERSTAND THE LAWS OF WELLNESS!!! Unfortunately too many people do not see weight gain as immediately life threatening. All overweight people admit they should lose weight but too often bypass the mental awareness of the life shortening potential of being overweight. Why do people have to be ill or dying to start taking care of themselves? You earn your health and longevity by the choices you make. Disease ... or being overweight ... that you develop in your lifetime is not bad luck!!!

Knowing how your immune system works helps you better understand how to boost it with an organic diet, herbs, natural based supplements and homeopathy. **Your immune system is your body's defense program designed to disrupt foreign agents that come into your body.** Your immune system recognizes the threat of invading bacteria and viruses that are looking for a place to breed ... *and because this would be at the expense of your body balance, your immune system eliminates or neutralizes the culprit.*

Most people will not escape getting the flu one or more times during their lifetime. There is a 'flu season', but it can strike anyone, anytime during the year. For most people it is a relatively short period of misery. For others it can be incredibly serious requiring hospitalization ... even death as the outcome. Your body comes with a 'flu shield' called the *IMMUNE SYSTEM.* **THE TRICK TO TREATING THE FLU**

IS TO PREVENT IT!!! If your body is healthy, it can survive an outbreak in your home, your work or your community.

Since it is not easy to penetrate the body's natural defense in the first place, your immune system knows the foreign agent is strong enough to break through the antibacterial and antiviral properties in the sinus, throat and nasal mucous membranes. The acid condition in the stomach can also kill organisms that get past the mucous membranes. Mucous, tears, saliva and other body fluids wash away most microorganisms. If it gets past those, a fever offers an unsuitable environment for the organism to live. **NEVER SUPPRESS A HARD WORKING FEVER UNLESS IT IS LIFE THREATENING!** If you want to take something for a slight to moderate fever, check with your health food store about Ferrum Phos., a natural cell salt that helps your body handle the invasion.

The main line of defense in your immune system is the cells that fight infection. They rush to the infected spot, engulf the intruding organism and destroy it by consuming and digesting it:

1. **B CELLS** – Growing out of your bone marrow, B Cells produce protein antibodies that stop the foreign agents dead in their tracks.

2. **T CELLS** – Grow in your thymus gland and are primarily responsible for making cells immune to viruses. They secrete certain molecules that attract other immune cells to come to the place of infection, and the *T Cells act as managers for all the defensive activity.* T Cells are always circulating … always on the lookout for anything out of the ordinary.

3. **KILLER T CELLS** – They have a one track mind … to wipe out the foreign invader. They bind to the foreign invader and release enzymes that kill it. It is the Killer T Cells that have to be inactivated in organ transplants.

4. **HELPER T CELLS** – They act as switch operators, flipping the switch so the immune response starts moving

and set the B Cells in motion. A great percentage of T Cells are Helper T Cells and are the ones targeted by HIV, making the body vulnerable to infection.

5. **SUPPRESSOR T CELLS** – These cells make sure the body does not get carried away with all the activity and regulate the immune response by adjusting or varying the intensity as needed.

6. **NATURAL KILLER CELLS** – They are your body's greatest weapon against infection and disease. They have free range throughout the body, with the ability to recognize and kill any foreign invader upon contact.

Your entire immune system is a series of checks and balances, with every defensive measure needing to be triggered by something, and then backed up by another defense.

TRY RUNNING THAT COMPLICATED SYSTEM WITH A DONUT AND COFFEE FOR BREAKFAST!!!

The incredibly important immune cells are the **front lines** of the immune response. In the **back lines** the organs that collectively make up the 'lymph system' include the bone marrow, thymus, spleen, tonsils and lymph nodes that are sprinkled throughout the body. *When you have an infection, the closest lymph node will swell up to contain the toxins.*

The immune system functions on its own without your conscious help. However, it needs to be kept healthy like your heart, bones or any other organ or system in your body. **The stress to the immune system is monumentally greater than it was even 50 years ago.** *Today … living in modern America … we need to make better choices to take some stress off the immune system, so it is there when we need it. Eating* **organic food** *and drinking* **filtered, energized water** *is a no-brainer in modern America.* **Daily exercise** *improves circulation allowing the T and B Cells to arrive on the scene of an infection quickly and put it down before it begins to multiply and cause you symptoms.*

Now look at your body and say, "Thank you immune system for all

your hard work … and I'll take better care of you now." **Little things collectively make a big difference like showering at night so your bed is not full of dust mites that produce allergic responses and make your adrenals work all night instead of resting. And do not forget to thump your thymus gland on your breastbone 3-4 times a day. Be good to your body and your body will protect you!!!**

Most people today have heard of the term 'autoimmune disease.' I've had three medical doctors in my office say about 60% of the patients they see in their offices have an autoimmune disease. *What is it, and why it is becoming so common in modern America?* You just read above how strong the immune system is against foreign invaders. Imagine what could happen if the immune system started attacking its own body's cells. In an autoimmune disease the immune system mistakenly attacks its own body and targets cells, tissues and organs that are not foreign at all. **This happens when the overworked immune system works so hard to deal with your needs, that it makes *mistakes.***

I am constantly reading articles that say we have much to learn about autoimmune disease … scientists are trying to find therapies that work on the body's immune response … ultimately science hopes to find ways to prevent autoimmune diseases. I also read articles 30 years ago that said we could stop cancer. The reality of politics is that research and the ultimate cure using drugs are more of a focus then the **simple rules of health** that encourage **body balance.**

I suggest you look closely at the following suggestions that encourage your body not to make antibodies or deal with prolonged stress of needing to make antibodies daily:

1. *Reduce* dust mites in your bed with a barrier cloth cover for your mattress and pillow, no animals on or in the bed, clean bedding weekly and shower anytime from after dinner to bedtime.

2. *Drink* your healthy energized water daily, instead of juices that may contain mold requiring your adrenals to make antibodies. Juice, coffee and sodas have become America's

water … and that can lead to body stress … that leads to disease.

3. ***Eliminate*** dairy products and beef because America's obsession with dairy and beef requires the production of daily antibodies. Save dairy and beef for special or social occasions and not as part of your daily diet at home.

4. ***Eliminate*** any other protein based food to which you have a known allergic reaction, or suspect a problem because you crave a food and generally do not feel well. **Suspect the food you always choose when you do not feel well.**

5. ***Exercise*** daily selecting walking type exercise that encourages the lymphatic system to clean up foreign invaders and take the stress off the immune system.

6. ***Reduce*** your exposure to chemicals through your consumer purchasing power!!! No one knows the imbalance that can result from our obsessive use of chemicals in our food, drinks, clothing, bedding, air pollution, etc., etc., etc. AND NO ONE KNOWS WHAT HAPPENS IN THE BODY FROM THE NEW CHEMICAL COMBINATIONS PRODUCED FROM THE COLLECTION OF CHEMICALS INGESTED, INHALED, OR ABSORBED.

7. ***Understand*** that body balance is impossible if your urine and saliva is chronically imbalanced.

I COULD *REVIEW* ALL THE PREVIOUS INFORMATION THAT WOULD COLLECTIVELY HELP YOUR IMMUNE SYSTEM BE LESS LIKELY TO *GO CRAZY … AND ATTACK YOUR OWN BODY*. THIS IS WHY ALL THE INFORMATION IN THIS BOOK IS SO IMPORTANT. ENJOY YOUR ENERGETIC … HEALTHIER … SLIMMER BODY … NATURALLY!!!

WEIGHT LOSS TIP #25

SUMMARY

"The greatest advances in medicine have not been the discovery of new technology ... but in prevention."

-Health Financial Management Journal, June 1990

Correct nutrition produces energy ... and ENERGY is the fountain of youth ... AND THE SECRET TO WEIGHT CONTROL! Americans often believe that a single drug, or technological procedure, or a trip to the vitamin shop can cure a disease or heal the body. Overweight Americans count calories and measure food religiously and generally lose weight ... but too often gain it back. *Too many people blame hereditary weaknesses for everything.* However, all organs increase their level of activity in an attempt to compensate for the lowered activity of the weakest ones. For example, if you do not exercise ... the liver, kidneys and skin work harder. In doing so, they all use more of the nutrients available, and the whole body tends to become depleted.

Each organ obtains the nutrients it needs from the bloodstream ... **if** the nutrients are there based on the quality of what was eaten ... and digested ... and assimilated (food changed into a form the body can use). **IT ALL STARTS WITH WHAT YOU CHOOSE TO PUT INTO YOUR MOUTH!!!** You cannot digest and assimilate healthy nutrients if the nutrients were not **first** in the food you ate. Processed, chemically loaded, and refined food fills the stomach ... but our health statistics suggest not enough nutrients get to the cells. *New and improved* only refers to the bank accounts of the food producers and distributors ... **you**

cannot improve on Nature. *The typical American diet has become disease producing. On a recent trip, my husband and I stopped for gas early in the morning, and a man came out of the store with an extra large container of a soda and a bag of potato chips. Another day we were walking to a church early in the morning, and a man come out of a restaurant with a cup of coffee in one hand and an ice cream bar in the other.* **JUST BECAUSE YOU ARE NOT HUNGRY DOES NOT MEAN YOU HAVE CELLULAR HEALTH. WHEN YOU EAT ... THE FOOD MUST HAVE THE NUTRITIONAL VALUE NEEDED BY THE CELLS!!!**

It is time we stop and think about the fact that the majority of the world population dies prematurely from diseases that develop due to nutritional deficiencies in the diet. That puts a whole new perspective on the subject of nutrition that could be a new approach for most Americans struggling with fatigue, disease and weight gain. *There is no substitute for proper nutrition and no therapy or healing art that can keep a malnourished body free of disease.* Do not waste an opportunity to '*feed your cells.*' First, buy organic so the food might actually have the nutrients you expect in the food. The average housewife peels her vegetables, throwing away nutrients; then the food may be boiled and drained of even more nutrients or nuked in the microwave. **Treat your organic fruits and vegetables with respect for their life giving properties. Know that you are hydrated with energized water and your pH is in the normal range!**

We are what we eat ... and we also are what we do not eat. The body molds to the foods we put into it ... for better or for worse. Poor food habits that result in nutrient deficiencies in the brain could produce mild to bizarre misbehavior ... or something as simple as low motivation that does not bring out your best strengths. *Poor nutrition is often at the root of undeveloped or underdeveloped talents ... and this frustration can lead to overeating.* **YOU ARE SO LUCKY TO HAVE ALL THE BASIC KNOWLEDGE THAT CAN CHANGE THE QUALITY OF YOUR LIFE FROM MOTIVATION TO LOOKING GOOD IN A SWIMSUIT... ENJOY IT!!!**

Take your basic knowledge of wellness and add one more word ... **COMMITMENT.** The definition of commitment is ... to bind as by a promise; pledge. Welcome to a world where you can help yourself and be a mentor to raise the standards of those around you. **Stay focused … and realize you are reading this book for one reason … YOU DESERVE MORE!!! IF THE WORD 'CHANGE' IS UNCOMFORTABLE FOR YOU THEN ANOTHER WORD FOR CHANGE IS GROWTH**. *We are on earth for two reasons:*

- **To learn and grow.**

- **To be in service to mankind.**

Albert Einstein said the definition of insanity is, *"Doing the same thing every day and expecting a different result."* **IF WHAT YOU ARE DOING IS NOT WORKING FOR YOU, THEN DO SOMETHING DIFFERENT!!!**

In her book "THERE'S A HOLE IN MY SIDEWALK: THE ROMANCE OF SELF-DISCOVERY," Portia Nelson talks about changes. She demonstrates this through her poem discussing how she falls into a deep hole in the sidewalk multiple times and feels helpless thinking it's not her fault. Finally she pretends not to see the hole, but still falls in the hole believing it is still not her fault. When she falls in again, she accepts responsibility that it is her fault. She finally decides to walk around the hole … and then decides to walk down another street.

This anonymous quote states "getting something done is an accomplishment; getting something done right is an achievement."

After finishing my book you have the knowledge to do something right (achievement) by walking down another street. You can decide to make choices that support body balance. *You can decide to be more than slimmer … you can decide to be healthier and stay slim.* You can decide to be in control of your health on all levels of mental, emotional and physical. You can take responsibility for the outcome of your life. This book can change your mindset so you do not have to wait for the next crisis.

A quote by William James states "It is our attitude at the beginning of a difficult undertaking which, more than anything else, will determine its successful outcome."

People who are overweight are often imprisoned with some sense of security. This negative security can hold them prisoner in their subconscious mind even though their conscious mind desires weight loss. We have an opportunity to unleash the chains of negativism unless you are secure in your negative thinking, like in this Charles Dickens story;

> *Charles Dickens wrote about a man who had been in prison for many years and longed for freedom from his dungeon of despair and hopelessness. Finally, the day of his liberation arrived. He was led from his gloomy cell into the bright and beautiful world. He momentarily gazed into the sunlight, then turned and walked back to his cell. He had become so comfortable with confinement, the thought of freedom was overwhelming. For him the chains of darkness and despair were secure.*

Is the thought of change frightening for you? Freedom comes only to those who are willing to surrender the security of conscious or subconscious imprisonment. We do not always consciously admit what drives our thoughts and choices. If what you are doing is working for you then you may be in control of your conscious and subconscious thoughts. But if what you're doing is not working for you then mental (thinking) and emotional (feeling) may be more important than your physical needs in your weight loss program.

A very real problem within all of us can be the dread of discouragement. There are four main pitfalls of discouragement:

1. Discouragement can hurt your self-image. This negative thinking can set you up for making poor choices.

2. Discouragement causes us to see ourselves as less than we really are. This is the same as self-worth.

3. Discouragement causes us to blame others for our own state of health. This blame can be from spouse, pregnancies, relatives … everyone is to blame except self.

4. Discouragement causes us to blur the facts. We get so used

to our situation that how it all got started gets lost in the process.

Perseverance becomes the essence of your character and your character becomes the essence of hope. Great works are performed not by strength but by perseverance.

This quote by Jacob A. Riis is a good example of perseverance.

"When nothing seems to help, I go and look at a stone cutter hammering away at his rock. Perhaps a hundred times without as much as a crack showing in it. Yet, at the hundred and first blow, it will split in two, and I know it was not that blow that did it, but all that had gone before."

WEIGHT LOSS IS NOT JUST A CHALLENGE … IT IS A LIFE CHALLENGE!

In analyzing your effort, you need to accept the obvious from this quote by Glen Van Ekeren.

"The tough thing about learning self-discipline is that we need self-discipline in order to learn it."

Weight gain is not just an inconvenience. This is your life … it is not a rehearsal … and your life is an expression of your thoughts. Your thoughts determine your success in everything you do from what you eat, your daily activity, your attitude about your challenges, and your determination to succeed. There are actually two kinds of success. The very rare kind is a person who is just plain a genius. Most of us do not fall into that category. Most of us achieve success because we simply are developing ordinary qualities to a more than ordinary degree. In the dictionary, success comes before work. But in life, work comes before success.

CONGRATULATIONS … YOU ARE NOW IN CHARGE!

**"All our dreams can come true – if we have
the courage to pursue them."**

-Walt Disney

WEIGHT LOSS MEAL PLANNING

WEIGHT LOSS MEAL PLANNING

"Identify your greatest fear and walk directly towards it."

-Eleanor Roosevelt

We are our worst enemy. Buying and eating obnoxious concoctions created by the food processing industry creates an impossible situation for the human digestive tract that was never designed to digest. The typical American diet is disease producing. Life expectancy statistics in this country is expected to go down due to a nation that is overweight and struggling with chronic and acute illness.

We cannot blame the Western diet for our shocking disease statistics. We must accept the blame when we **choose** to eat nutritionally deprived and chemically loaded food. **You can refuse to eat the typical Western diet and pick real food instead of chemical food. You can take natural herbs, supplements derived from natural foods and use Homeopathic remedies to raise your constitutional ability to maintain wellness. These choices help you to enjoy dramatic health improvements in a shockingly short period of time.**

Why are we as Americans being treated to **live** with a problem and not taught how to **change** the problem? I read weight loss books with recipes containing many ingredients that can **contribute** to body imbalance and sabotage a permanent weight loss effort. Meal planning takes some understanding at first, but can quickly be routine when you learn what foods help you stay healthy and slim … and what foods cause many health problems. *Do not fear dietary changes. Just learn the principles of wellness and the body does the rest!*

- *Keep in mind the information on nightshade foods. At least for one whole* **month** *eliminate those foods if you have chronic or acute joint pain ... and then decide if you feel better.*

- *Keep in mind the information on salicylate foods. At least for one whole* **month** *eliminate those foods if you were hyperactive as a child and still find it hard to feel calm, cannot tolerate aspirin, perfume or smoke ... and then decide if you feel better.*

- *At least for one whole week eliminate dairy and beef products if you have chronic sinus or throat symptoms, frequent headaches or migraines, or* **any** *unexplained chronic or acute symptom* **anywhere** *in the body including the ever popular chronic fatigue and chronic muscle pain ... and decide if you feel better. Dairy and beef are not just in food. Your supplements and prescription drugs could contain dairy and/or beef ingredients. When in doubt have a compounding pharmacy formulate your prescription drugs in vegetarian capsules and fillers, and only buy supplements in vegetable capsules.*

- *At least for one whole month eliminate soy products if you have any signs of a hormone imbalance for women, history of fibroids or hormone receptive cancer, prostate symptoms for men or have been eating mostly non-organic food. Soy products contain phyto-estrogens that can add to estrogen build up in the body and may not always cause conscious symptoms but can contribute to an overall sense of poor health.*

- *At least for one whole month eliminate high fructose foods if you have belly fat, pre-diabetes or diabetes, or* **any** *chronic symptom that could be in part due to an unhealthy liver that has turned fructose into fat. Fructose could also be the cause of* intestinal symptoms both diarrhea and constipation ... and decide if you feel better.

–   *At least for six whole months make dietary choices* that help you towards your goal of having your clothes fit less tight. You may not lose weight at first because fat may be turning into muscle and muscle weighs more than fat. The weight loss will come if you stick to your determination to have a body that works in optimum performance.

–   *At least for six whole months have a plan to help you reach your best weight.* It may take longer than that but in six months you should know if you are making choices from a good plan. To determine your best weight take the inches above 60 and multiply by 5, add 110 for women and 120 for men. Example, you are 5 foot 2 inches, so multiply 2 x 5 = 10 plus 110 so your weight should be 120.

–   *At least for now accept that you are in school to learn about health.* Vegetables are **less** alkalizing when cooked, processed or canned as they lose vital minerals and enzymes. Steaming vegetables is better than boiling them. Drink the liquid that contains many nutrients with either choice of cooking. The greenest vegetables are the most alkalizing. Each day you can learn something interesting that will help you live healthier in our stressful world. ***ENJOY THE JOURNEY!!!***

–   *At least start to understand the quality of food that supports the best digestion.* Whole grains that are processed are more acidifying. For best digestion consume only **sprouted organic** whole grains. ***AGAIN, ENJOY THE JOURNEY OF ASSUMING RESPONSIBILTY FOR YOUR HEALTH THROUGH THE CHOICES YOU MAKE.***

–   *At least understand how to decide the best food choices based on your urine and saliva pH readings.* Meat and eggs are acid forming and should be eliminated until you *improve a very acidic system. If you must eat these foods with an acidic system make sure you eat 3-4 servings of alkalizing vegetables, or consider alkalizing supplements like Sun Chlorella daily. Sprouted organic bread is **less acidic** and **easier to digest** than regular bread.*

– *At least understand that proteins, fats and oils are not the problem in weight control. To eat a serious diet for weight loss you should give up all grains, fruit, fruit juice, refined sugar, and desserts made with high glycemic ingredients. The diet of easy to digest proteins and vegetables will produce the best weight loss. Know your ability to digest food is controlled by your urine pH (stress) and saliva pH (digestion). Become familiar with the website* www.glycemicindex.com *to find those foods under 55 that help in your meal planning.*

Once you start feeling better with more energy and less chronic symptoms your weight will start to normalize naturally. What you tried for a few weeks or months will easily become your lifetime routine. Once you learn the basic principles of wellness you will have the knowledge to get off the disease merry-go-round. People on the disease merry-go-round will never get off with the traditional approach to the treatment of disease or weight loss. Symptoms do not suggest you are deficient in a drug. What a symptom does suggest is that you are nutritionally deficient, in toxic overload, and your constitutional ability to stay well (your Vital Force) is down. It is up to you to learn how to heal little nagging chronic symptoms with the principles of wellness so you are not forced to treat a health crisis!

Let's start with what you should have in your kitchen …

MUST HAVE KITCHEN EQUIPMENT

SLOW COOKER (ALSO CALLED CROCK POT)

GEORGE FOREMAN GRILL

SMALL CAST IRON GRILL

LARGE SKILLET WITH A LID FOR STIR FRY RECIPES (now a favorite)

LARGE FLAT GRIDDLE FOR FRENCH TOAST AND PANCAKES (made with low glycemic grains and Coconut Nectar)

PRESSURE COOKER

LARGE SOUP KETTLE (now a favorite)

HEAVY DUTY BLENDER (blender drinks give you the best nutrition and are time saving)

HAND MIXER

OVERSIZED RICE COOKER FOR COMPLETE DINNERS (you can make any stew in this that does not have to contain rice. Substitute Red Inca Quinoa for the high glycemic rice.)

SMALL VEGETABLE CHOPPER

TOASTER (lower glycemic index Millet bread tastes better toasted)

SMALL COUNTER TOP OVEN IS OK BUT NO MICROWAVE!!!

Dori Luneski, R.N., N.D.

INVEST IN AT LEAST ONE GOOD SHARP KNIFE

INVEST IN A GOOD SET OF STAINLESS STEEL COOKWARE

QUESADILLA MACHINE AND/OR WAFFLE MAKER
   (invaluable once you adjust your recipes to be low glycemic)

*A SET OF LOCKING REFRIGERATOR CONTAINERS (check
   with QVC)*

*A good place to look for kitchen ware is QVC. Check online at QVC. COM or on your TV. You can call Customer Service 1-800-367-9444 to find the next TV show on kitchen products. Many cooking pots and pans are coated with a non stick surface that originally scratched easily. Non-stick surfaces today are harder and healthier. **I recommend you throw out any old pans that have a scratched surface.** Stainless steel, glass or cast iron is still a better choice.*

MUST HAVE BASIC INGREDIENTS

MAKE YOUR OWN BETTER BUTTER – *with a hand mixer or food processor mix 1 cup of water and 1 cup of any tolerated **mild tasting** organic oil (like Spectrum brand of canola that is organic) with 1 pound of VERY SOFT organic butter (salted or unsalted your choice) until completely creamy.* Olive oil is not a good choice for Better Butter because the taste compromises the flavor of the butter. Butter does not have the allergic protein properties of milk because butter is made only from the milk fat. Butter is high in Vitamin A and Vitamin D, and Better Butter should be considered a healthy spread. You should store Better Butter in the refrigerator in a covered container. Do not use Better Butter in any bake recipe as the added water could negatively alter the expected result.

*Allergic to eggs?** Many recipes work well with the following substitutes:

– *1 tablespoon of organic sprouted flaxseed and 2 tablespoons of water for each egg. If you are making French Toast just add more nondairy milk and forget the water.*

– *2 tablespoons of arrowroot flour to the recipe = 1 egg*

– *See directions on the Ener-G Egg Replacer box.*

*Look for the products from Coconut Secret** in your health food store. The products are made from the sap of the tree and do not have a coconut flavor. Each product is organic, gluten and dairy free, soy free, has a low glycemic index of 35 and are enzymatically alive mineral rich food choices. The Coconut Aminos can be used like soy sauce for flavor on any protein, in any recipe and salad dressings. The low glycemic, low fructose Coconut Nectar can be used in place of organic maple syrup. The Coconut Crystals can be a substitute for refined brown or white sugar in the same proportions. The Coconut Vinegar may be a great substitute for grain or apple cider vinegar if you have a problem with those foods. If you cannot find these awesome products call (888)-369-3393 or www.coconutsecret.com.

*Imagine brand Butternut Squash soup is soy free and is a staple you can use many times added to soups and stews, or just heat a cup of this delicious soup for part of a quick meal or hot drink.

*For people allergic to chicken and eggs a must staple is the **Imagine brand organic No-Chicken broth.**

*Quinoa is a gluten-free, easy to digest **complete** protein grain that should be a staple in every kitchen. Use quinoa **flakes** in blender drinks. You can cook the "bird seed" version of quinoa like rice using either white quinoa seeds or the product called Red Inca. You can also cook quinoa **flakes** as a cereal and top with whatever nuts or seeds you like, plus a non-dairy unsweetened milk and a low glycemic index sweetener like Coconut Crystals or Coconut Nectar. Quinoa flakes is the perfect food to stretch any soup or stew recipe and add protein; and Quinoa flour is the perfect food to thicken any recipe. This stir-fry recipe example is high in antioxidants and nutrients:

Cook 1 cup washed Red Inca Quinoa with 2 cups of water or broth and stir-fry with natural sea salt and 1 teaspoon of sesame oil. Add 1/2 cup finely diced scallions, leeks or mild medium chopped white onion, 4 very large minced garlic cloves and 1/4 cup finely chopped organic carrots. You can be creative and add chopped celery, chopped leaves of Bok Choy, fresh chopped herbs and/or chopped cabbage. Root vegetables like turnips or parsnips can be added … be creative and change each stir-fry. Cover and cook until liquid is absorbed for about 15–20 minutes. Toss with chopped fresh parsley (or dried if necessary). Garnish with broccoli sprouts … or add small pieces of fresh broccoli to the last few minutes of cooking.

THERE IS NO SET RECIPE FOR A STIR-FRY ... IT IS ONLY LIMITED BY YOUR IMAGINATION.

*Keep a stock supply of ...

- **organic canned beans** *for soups, recipes and salads. Learn to use Garbanzo beans (chick peas) that are low in saturated fat, cholesterol and sodium, and high in fiber and protein. Do not be discouraged if you get some gas when you first start to eat some beans. As your health improves, so will your digestion.* **Make sure you wash every bit of the foam off organic canned beans before using in any recipe.** *That foam is the indigestible sugar that causes digestive symptoms. High fiber diets may be a valuable benefit for both weight loss and high blood pressure.*

- **spelt** *(easier to digest than wheat but is a gluten grain) or corn (a non-gluten grain) tortillas you keep in the freezer and hard organic taco shells. Sprouted spelt bread is easier to digest than sprouted wheat. Look for sprouted spelt in the freezer section of your health food store.*

- **organic chicken broth**, *or non-chicken broth (that can be used in any recipe that calls for vegetable broth).*

- *unrefined, organic* **olive oil**.

- *organic* **sesame oil** *or other organic oil of choice. Keep in mind your suspected issues like salicylates that would be a problem with some oils like grapeseed.*

- *unrefined* **sea salt** *that still clumps and contains the moisture that holds the trace minerals. My favorite is Redmond Real Salt.*

- **organic dried herbs** *you store in the refrigerator. If you have the room and the interest start an herb garden that will add incredible taste treats to your recipes.* **Fresh herbs** *are nearly twice as strong in a recipe as dried herbs. You can buy small* *amounts of fresh herbs in most health food stores, but unless you grow your own, only buy one kind at a time. They will turn brown in the refrigerator and only last less than a week before they start to turn bad. Once you get use to adding them to nearly every recipe it is easier to clean up what you buy.*

— *low glycemic index and fructose free **sweetners** like **Stevia** that can be bitter unless you buy the highest quality. **Lo Han** is a Chinese fruit sugar that is not known to have any negative side effects. If you cannot find it where you shop you can order it from Vitacost.com and check the internet to learn all about the value of this sweet and healthy fruit. **Coconut Secret** products are low glycemic index. Learn to use Stevia for small needs like a blender drink or cup of tea, and use Coconut Crystals for baking substitution for refined sugar or brown sugar in equal amounts. Use Coconut Nectar for any recipe that calls for a liquid sweetener such as honey or agave in equal amounts. Not recommended is Agave because it is 100% fructose and Xylitol because it causes many people to have intestinal bloating.*

— *non-stick **olive oil** pan spray (does contain soy lecithin). If soy is a problem just use olive oil spread with a paper towel.*

— *easier to digest gluten free Tinkyada brand **rice pastas** that when cooked maintains the texture and taste of wheat pasta.*

— *sprouted organic whole grain soy free bread is found in the freezer section of health food stores. **Sprouted Spelt may be tolerated** by **some** gluten sensitive people. Keep all healthy whole grain bread in the freezer to store or in the refrigerator to use, NEVER in a bread drawer.*

— *organic **nut butters** and assorted organic **nuts and seeds**.*

— *fruit spread from organic companies that make **just fruit spreads** that will be lower in sugar than jams and jellies but still not a recommended food daily.*

- *assorted canned products that you use in salads like black or green olives, artichoke hearts, organic beets. Highly recommended are Terra Sticks that are root vegetables in sticks that add crunch to your salads (or make your own substitute by crumbling Terra Chips). Terra products are a delectable medley of exotic vegetables that do not have to say organic.*

- *wheat free gluten free flour choices like Quinoa, millet, coconut flour and whole grain Teff. Look for Bob's Red Mill flour selections for wonderful all natural products that should be basic stock ingredients if you have poor digestion or gluten intolerance. With some ingredient adjustments the recipes on the back of the Teff bag for cookies and muffins could add a spark to your diet. Look for EnerG products like Tapioca flour and see the recipe for tapioca on the box substituting non-dairy unsweetened milk and a low glycemic sweetener like Coconut Crystals for great tapioca pudding.*

- *non-dairy milk of choice should be unsweetened but may be made sweeter with Stevia or Coconut Crystals.*

- *organic whole grain cold cereals of choice, and hot cereals like Rice and Shine cream of rice. Quinoa flakes have a lower glycemic index and may be a better cereal at the start of a weight loss program. I do not recommend dried fruit on cereal because you tend to eat more dried fruit than you would the fresh fruit and that increases carbohydrates. Another problem is that dried fruit is high in mold content. If you want a little dried fruit on cereal you should rinse the choice well in warm water first to reduce the mold content. Sweeten cold or hot cereals with Coconut Crystals or Coconut Nectar. Coconut Nectar is very thick syrup that will pour easier if ¼ cup water is added to the whole bottle and mixed thoroughly before pouring. Mix cinnamon with Coconut Crystals as a sweetener or a spread for toast.*

- *organic salad dressings, or ingredients to make your own salad dressing like starting with a base of hummus ... and*

... whatever you want to make a great salad dressing. Keep organic bottled lemon juice to spark up many recipes or make salad dressing. Coconut Secret Vinegar is fabulous and is preferred for people sensitive to apple cider vinegar or balsamic (grape) vinegar.

- canned **LITE coconut milk** *you can use in cream sauces, pancakes, baking, smoothies and dozens of other recipes. Light coconut milk has 70% less saturated fat and adds a sweet, nutty richness to foods. Regular coconut milk should also be a staple because it is needed for any recipe that calls for half and half or whipping cream dairy products.*

- **canned fish** *for those quick meals or days you forget to thaw something for dinner. Bottled clam juice can be used often in many fish recipes. Add to Wild Caught Boiled Baby Clams in water for an easy low caloric dinner over Quinoa pasta. For favorite recipes considered Wild Caught Skinless and Boneless Sardines in water, low mercury tuna from sustainably caught **Wild Planet brand** of Albacore or Skipjack tuna or Alaskan salmon (in a BPA free can).*

- **whole grain rice** *choices. Some people who dislike the taste and texture of brown rice over white rice may be pleasantly surprised that organic whole grain Jasmine or Basmati rice tastes delicious and lighter.*

- **Sprouted products** *for the best digestion. If you are a senior like I am (78) or have poor digestion from an acidic pH or a lifetime of stress you should look for anything that is sprouted because those products are better digested. When I make soup or other recipes I use Sprouted Mung Beans, Sprouted Quinoa and Sprouted Lentils. Look for the truRoots brand and if you cannot find them check www.truroots.com*

- **assorted canned goods or ingredients** *that you need for your favorite recipes. Keep your pantry well stocked and you'll have what you need when the desire strikes. Do not forget* *organic canned pumpkin and organic canned sweet potatoes that have saved the flavor of many recipes for me.*

– *Dijon mustard or your favorite mustard can save many recipes. If you like a strong mustard, look for Roland 100% Organic Extra Strong Dijon mustard.*

Now that you have a basic idea of how to build a highly functioning kitchen, making a healthy meal in a short period of time should be a lot easier. Some people like to cook and others do not. Not liking to cook should not mean you do not eat well. If you do not have time to shop weekly then make the one shopping trip a month be big enough to stock your cupboard and freezer for a month. **Learning how to shop is as important as learning how to prepare meals.**

If you eat healthy food and digest your food you will FEED YOUR CELLS AND HAVE LESS CRAVINGS BECAUSE YOU ARE NOT IN CELLULAR STARVATION! Simple meals can be delicious, nutritious and healthy if they contain organic, chemical free choices.

The following **IDEAS** are not written up as recipes. Many people look at new recipes and still go back to what is familiar because they do not have the time or energy to learn something new. **IDEAS** however spark an interest in creating a new twist on an old favorite, or remind you of a meal suggestion you used to eat.

The recipes that are included in this book are easy to fix and do not contain numerous ingredients that you have to buy to prepare … and may not use again for a long time. Because money is usually tight in any family, it is a waste of your time to read a lot of recipes that require you to buy a number of ingredients you will not use often. These recipes are all easy basic family meals you will turn to often when life gets hectic. **You should have IDEAS for quick meals that do not include any foods you now suspect should be avoided.**

BREAKFAST IDEAS

- Take an organic **grapefruit or pear** and section it into bite size pieces in a dish. If you do not suspect salicylate foods are a problem you could section an orange or any seasonal low fructose fruit like berries. Top with a few organic sunflower and pumpkin seeds, or your favorite chopped organic nut. Completely stir in a low glycemic index and fructose free sweetener until dissolved like Stevia or Coconut Nectar or Coconut Crystals. You can add a little non-dairy unsweetened milk if desired.

- Whole grains are mucus forming, but if sinus symptoms are not your problem you might enjoy cooked organic oatmeal (if you do not have a gluten grain problem). Cooked gluten free **Cream of Rice or cooked Quinoa flakes** are both easier to digest than cooked wheat. Add a little **Sprouted** Flaxseed for added nutrition. Top with a low glycemic index sweetener like Coconut Crystals and your choice of non-dairy unsweetened milk. You can thin cooked cereal with more water or non-dairy unsweetened milk and put into a container to drink on your way to work or on a trip.

- Cut up an **organic apple (if you do not suspect a salicylate problem) or pear** into quarters and spread each quarter with your favorite nut butter or peanut butter. This can be fixed at home and eaten on the way to work or when you get to work.

- Heat one tablespoon of **Lewis Laboratory Brewers Yeast Buds** (that is not from a yeast base) in a cup of carob or chocolate rice milk to make a delicious hot drink. Make toast out of a tolerated bread and spread Better Butter and a mix of cinnamon and Coconut Crystals on the toast. Millet bread is available in health food stores for people who are gluten intolerant. Sprouted spelt bread in the freezer section of health food stores is easier to digest than wheat breads. If you are trying to lower estrogen levels because of a history of fibroids or cancer make sure if you decide to eat a sprouted wheat bread that is does not contain sprouted soybeans.

- Put two organic brown rice cakes in the toaster to crisp and top with your **favorite nut butter or peanut butter.** You can also crisp rice cakes in the oven at 300 degrees for five minutes. Even freshly opened rice cakes will be crispier if slightly heated.

- A serving of your favorite **low fructose fruit** along with a handful of your favorite nut mix is a quick breakfast, mid morning or afternoon snack.

- Put Better Butter on two toasted organic sprouted bread slices then cut into one inch cubes. Place into a bowl and top with two organic **soft cooked eggs** and natural sea salt.

- Keep organic **hard boiled eggs** in the refrigerator to eat anytime you are in a hurry or want a snack. Eat peeled hard boiled eggs anytime with or without added sea salt.

- Buying **Polenta** made from corn in the health food store is easier than making your own. Slice and warm in Better Butter, **very** lightly drizzle with Coconut Nectar, and top with seeds or chopped nuts.

- The old standby unsweetened **dry cereal** is always a quick breakfast but make sure the choice is organic and a tolerated whole grain. Top with any non-dairy unsweetened milk and sweeten with Coconut Crystals. You can sprinkle dry cereal with sunflower and pumpkin seeds or **Sprouted** Flaxseeds for extra nutrition. Dry cereal can also be made sweeter by adding your fresh seasonal fruit for the day. Because of our fast paced lifestyle, dry cereal has become a way of life in modern America. However, processing reduces or eliminates some nutrients and proteins so only choose dry cereal in a time crunch.

- **French toast** using tolerated grains can be delicious without eggs by using 1 tablespoon of Sprouted Flaxseed per egg added to non-dairy unsweetened milk, sea salt and cinnamon. Top with Better Butter and add a tiny drizzle of Coconut Nectar.

- **Scrambled eggs** will be lighter if you add 1 tablespoon of any non-dairy unsweetened milk or water per egg, pinch of sea salt, and low heat scramble in Better Butter in a sprayed skillet. Most people think of toast as being two slices, but you can cut calories with just one slice when served with eggs. Make scrambled eggs taste different with chopped turkey bacon or slices of organic turkey sausage.

- Left over homemade **muffins** (like the recipe you adjust on the back of the Teff package), pumpkin or zucchini bread or any other favorite recipe spread with Better Butter makes a quick breakfast choice.

- **Learn to take a favorite recipe and adjust the ingredients to be healthier like this Banana Bread. Remember to add or subtract amounts as desired to make it taste right to you. Every recipe can be an original!**

    -2 cups all-purpose flour change to Quinoa flour

    -1 ½ tsp. baking powder change to aluminum free

    -1/2 tsp baking soda

–½ tsp cinnamon should be organic

–1/4 tsp salt should be natural unrefined sea salt

–1/4 tsp. ground nutmeg should be organic

–1/8 tsp. ginger should be organic

–2 lightly beaten eggs should be organic

–1 ½ cups mashed very ripe bananas should be organic. This is a good recipe to make when the store has ripe bananas ½ price. Bananas are high in fructose but a special occasional recipe is a nice break from ordinary.

Experiment using shredded green or yellow zucchini instead of bananas. Always taste zucchini before using in a recipe as it can sometimes be bitter.

–1 cup sugar change to Coconut Crystals

–1/2 cup melted butter should be organic (not Better Butter due to extra water)

–1/3 cup chopped walnuts or pecans should be organic

Preheat oven to 350 degrees and grease a 9 inch loaf pan. Combine the first 7 ingredients. In a separate bowl combine the next 4 ingredients. Stir egg mixture into flour until moist but still lumpy and fold in nuts. Bake 50 minutes and cool completely before slicing.

– **The easiest, best digested, and most nutritious breakfast you can consume is a blender drink.** If you make a full quart drink you can drink ½ for breakfast and ½ for lunch. To regain your health you should drink blender drinks seven days a week. For maintenance you could reduce the drinks to five days a week, or just on work days. The follow amount is a quart drink for adults:

   * *24 ounces of filtered **water** with added electrolyte*

drops plus ½ cup of 100% pure **Coconut Water** (optional but very helpful for hydration and healthy blood plasma).

*   2 tablespoons of mixed **sunflower and pumpkin seeds**.

*   1 tablespoon **sesame seeds** that is a good food for the pancreas. **All nuts and seeds should be stored in the freezer.**

*   1/3 cup of **Quinoa flakes** located in the cereal section of a health food store. Quinoa is an easy to digest **complete** protein, gluten free and low glycemic index for weight control. Quinoa is available as flakes that can be cooked like cereal or used uncooked in drinks, and seeds that cook up like rice for any recipe. Quinoa flour can be used for anything from pancakes to breading to baking. **Quinoa is one of the best foods in your wellness program for digestion and nutrition.**

*   2 tablespoons of **ORGANIC SPROUTED Flaxseed.**

*   1 scoop of any non-dairy and soy free **protein powder**; or any vegetarian organic greens product such as **Greens Pak** or antioxidant product like **Reds Pak** available in health food stores or on line. For any product you cannot find check Amazon.com with free shipping over $25.00 or Vita Cost with free shipping over $50.00.

Read protein powder products carefully as some products contain gluten grains or other foods you may not tolerate.

*   You can add 2 tablespoons of Old Chatham **Sheep Yogurt or Goat Yogurt** for extra flavor and nutrition.

* *You can add 1 tablespoon Bob's Red Mill whole grain **Teff flour** for extra nutrition, stamina and helps to thicken the drink.*

* *You can add 2 nuts each of a selection of your tolerated **nuts** such as walnuts, Brazil nuts, pecans, cashews and/or Hazelnuts. Both nuts and seeds should be avoided if you experience nausea from possible problems with your gallbladder.*

* ***Optional foods** to add include pomegranate powder or beet powder.*

* *At this point you can **add the following liquid** to complete the quart 32 ounces: any tolerated non-dairy unsweetened milk, 100% pure pomegranate juice (not a blend), fresh grapefruit juice found in the fresh juice section and not the bottled juice section, any tolerated organic vegetable juice or a selection of fresh vegetables of choice.*

* *Sweeten with **Stevia or Coconut Crystals**.*

If you are too busy to make a blender drink, you can make a blender **shake** by adding only those ingredients that dissolve if you shake the container. This drink could be enough during a stressful day, or just a shopping trip.

- **Waffles** can be made gluten free with the Namaste waffle mix. Follow the recipe on the bag and consider adding blueberries to the batter. Also, Hodgson Mills Multi Purpose Flour is gluten free and has the advantage of not containing sugar so you can add Coconut Crystals. For either of the above options, if you cannot eat eggs, and can tolerate potato starch, substitute EnerG Egg Replacer for the eggs. Top with Better Butter and drizzle with Coconut Nectar. For a fancy treat, you can make a blueberry compote:

    To 1 cup of water, add 2 TBPS cornstarch, ¼ tsp sea salt,

1 tsp cinnamon, and 2 TBSP Coconut Crystals. Cook until thickened for two minutes. Add 1 bag organic frozen blueberries (not thawed) and cook on low heat for ten minutes. Adjust salt and Coconut Crystals to taste as blueberries can vary in sweetness; add more water if it cooks too thick. This is fabulous over waffles, pancakes, and can be used as a substitute for high sugar jams on toast.

– **Pancakes** can be made low glycemic and easier to digest by using Quinoa for the flour. This recipe is a winner … and will also make crisp waffles because of the whipped egg whites. For a soft waffle, stir in the eggs and do not beat the egg whites:

*Mix together 1 cup of Quinoa flour, 1 cup of Original Rice Milk OR water, 1 tablespoon organic mild flavored oil (like Canola), 1 tablespoon Coconut Nectar (needed to brown the pancakes), 2 teaspoons aluminum free baking powder and 2 hormone and antibiotic free egg yolks. Whip the 2 egg whites until stiff peaks and fold into mixture with a spoon. With a large ladle put batter onto a preheated and oiled griddle. Top with Better Butter and **drizzle lightly** with Coconut Nectar. If you want to reduce the sugar you can top your pancakes with Better Butter and cinnamon, or add a few blueberries to the batter (or consider the blueberry compote recipe above). You can also add some chopped nuts to the batter for added nutrition. **There is a big difference between saying drizzle lightly instead of flooding the pancakes with syrup. Learning to cut down on syrups may make it possible not to eliminate your favorite foods like 100% pure Maple Syrup.***

– You are what you eat so pay attention to how you react to foods mentally and physically. *Long term symptoms can sometimes be so masked you do not know if you can tolerate a food. Suspect any food you eat most often … your food choice if you are hungry … and will go to the grocery store at inconvenient times to make sure you have it … as possible causes of your chronic symptoms.*

LUNCH OR DINNER IDEAS

- **Corn, spelt or brown rice tortillas** filled with organic canned refried black or pinto beans, sprouts or chopped organic lettuce, chopped white onion (less strong than red or yellow onions), diced ripe avocado and shredded Manchego sheep cheese. You can also use the same ingredients without the lettuce and grill in a Quesadilla machine.

- **Polenta** is cooked corn meal found in health food stores and is a gluten free food that can be sliced, warmed and topped with Better Butter and Coconut Nectar. It can also be topped with organic applesauce if you are not sensitive to salicylate foods and that is considered your one fruit for the day.

- If you took the time to make **soup** for the freezer, you have a quick lunch or dinner for many meals. You can stretch most soup by adding organic chicken broth (or Imagine no chicken broth) and organic refried pinto beans or any other canned organic bean. Organic turkey parts or ground turkey, whole chicken, turkey bacon or sausage, less expensive cuts of lamb, or buffalo cuts are all examples of the stock base for soup. From there use your imagination and what is in the refrigerator or cupboard. Besides all the legumes you can add canned pumpkin or canned sweet potatoes. Clean up root vegetables or any other vegetable you want to use up and know it is time to make soup. My soup is never from a recipe but it is always good and when my freezer shelf gets low I make more. For quick thawing at the last minute just put the frozen soup into an oven casserole with a lid in the oven at 400 degrees for 30 minutes or until heated. Heating in the oven eliminates the worry of scorching the soup on the stove.

- **Leftover chicken (or turkey** if you are allergic to chicken and eggs) make great lunch salads or sandwiches. If you want to reduce or eliminate grains you can made a sandwich like roll with a large leaf of romaine lettuce.

- Unsalted, organic corn or rice chips can be covered with chopped green onions, chopped olives, sliced cherry tomatoes (if tolerated),and shredded Manchego sheep cheese; melt in a 350 degree oven for a **healthy nachos** treat.

- Make your own low-fat **sausage** with any hormone and antibiotic free **ground meat** like turkey, chicken, buffalo, lamb or ostrich by adding natural sea salt and sage to taste. Only add organic fresh ground black pepper (if you do not suspect nightshade foods) at the table, because ground pepper can turn rancid and cooked black pepper is hard on the liver.

- **Wild Planet Sardines in water should be considered one of the best foods you can eat.** I attribute eating sardines daily for a year with its high ability to regenerate cells as the reason for being able to walk again after 20 years of Lupus. Fix it any way you like … but make it a part of your diet! Mix in the same way you would mix tuna fish and top mixture onto organic rice crackers or organic rice cakes crisped in the toaster. If you are avoiding grains wrap in Romaine lettuce. Heat with Butternut Squash soup, add to a salad with your favorite dressing, add to Manchego sheep cheese for a grilled cheese sandwich, or an ingredient on a Quesadilla. Not all brands of sardines taste the same. Before you give up on this super food try the Wild Planet brand.

- If you do not have a problem with the nightshade paprika, organic chicken and turkey **hot dogs** can be good eaten with organic lettuce or washed sprouts, chopped onions or whatever you like. If you have a problem with grains, wrap the basic ingredients in a large Romaine lettuce leaf or Chinese cabbage leaf.

- Turn left over coleslaw into a base for **tacos** that is only limited by your imagination. Coleslaw is easy to make if you have a small food chopper. I love my Quisinart brand and use it constantly. First layer slaw on top of flat corn or spelt tortillas that you have warmed on a skillet or in the oven, and top with any leftover protein like chicken or fish, chopped organic lettuce and shredded Manchego sheep cheese. Roll up for a quick treat.

- Winter Squash Soup is a complicated and time consuming recipe and yet this soup is delicious. A quick version of this soup is to buy organic Imagine brand **Butternut Squash Soup** and heat for a great hot treat anytime. Add cinnamon for added flavor, sardines, or organic turkey or chicken hot dogs.

- A recommended snack lunch any day should be your favorite flavored **Hummus** from the health food store, and piled onto an organic rice cracker that is easier to digest than wheat crackers. You can toast rice cakes in the toaster for one minute to crisp and spread with Hummus. Chickpeas in Hummus is a near perfect food! Regular Hummus or Roasted Garlic Hummus makes a fabulous base for salad dressings by thinning with olive oil, Coconut Vinegar and Coconut Crystals or Nectar. Add water if still too thick. Spectrum brand of Canola Mayonnaise makes another flavor treat with the Hummus base.

- A lower carbohydrate quick version of **grilled cheese** is to lightly spread your favorite mustard and Better Butter over **one** slice of a tolerated sprouted grain bread and cover with slices of Manchego Sheep Cheese … then broil until melted.

— Peel and mash an **avocado** with lemon or lime juice, plain sheep or goat yogurt (optional), tomato and/or cucumber if tolerated, and onion or garlic if desired. Pile onto an endive or Chinese cabbage leaf.

— This fabulous recipe of **Quinoa Crackers** can stand alone as a light snack or lunch:

> *Preheat oven to 400 degrees. In a medium bowl mix together 1 ½ cup quinoa flour, 1 level cup grated Manchego sheep cheese, 1 teaspoon garlic powder and ½ teaspoon baking soda. In a separate bowl whisk together 2 tablespoons olive oil, 3 tablespoons cold water, 1 large hormone and antibiotic free egg (or EnerG Egg replacer) and ½ teaspoon sea salt. Add dry ingredients to wet ingredients and stir until thoroughly combined. If dough appears dry and crumbly add 1 teaspoon of water at a time until it holds together. Divide the dough into halves and knead a few turns until a ball forms. Flour an area with quinoa flour and roll out the dough to 1/8 inch thickness using extra quinoa flour to prevent sticking. Repeat process with the remaining dough. Press 2 tablespoons hulled sesame seeds gently into the dough. Cut the dough into 2 inch squares with a pizza cutter. Bake until golden for 12–15 minutes. Store in an airtight container in the refrigerator. This is a dry cracker and may be enjoyed more topped with tuna fish or sardines, cut up hot dogs, turkey bologna, or any tolerated protein. Enjoy!!!*

DINNER MAIN COURSES

– **Pasta** is not always eliminated in a weight loss program. Eat smaller portions of the pasta and a large salad. Sometimes just a little of a favorite food can satisfy you. Pasta should be easy like this recipe that feeds 4:

* *Cook a small box or package of your choice of organic pasta in salted water until tender. Quinoa or Tinkyada brand of rice pasta is gluten free, lower in glycemic index, and easy to digest so consider this over wheat pasta.*

* *Heat 2 tablespoons of extra-virgin olive oil with 1 tablespoon of Better Butter, 2 tablespoons of fresh organic lemon juice, 4 large garlic cloves (or 2 teaspoons of fresh chopped garlic in jars), fresh or dried parsley and ½ teaspoon of natural sea salt. Add and cook 1 cup organic fresh or organic frozen vegetable of choice like broccoli or string beans for 2 minutes. Add to drained and thoroughly rinsed pasta to wash off the excess starch.*

* *Add 1/2 cup of thinly sliced fresh basil for the best flavor, or use dried organic basil to taste.*

* *Add ¼ cup of chopped walnuts or pecans*

* ***Shred over the top before serving*** *the desired amount of Manchego sheep cheese and enjoy with a healthy salad.*

– **Herb and Lemon Fish:**

> *Preheat oven to 425 degrees. Oil a baking dish with olive oil. Grate 1 teaspoon of just the very thin outer layer of a lemon, and then juice 1 tablespoon of lemon. Add to 1 tablespoon extra-virgin olive oil and ½ teaspoon organic thyme plus ½ teaspoon organic oregano. If you have fresh herbs use 1 teaspoon of each herb for a more vibrant flavor. Drizzle over fish of choice and bake for about 12-15 minutes depending on the thickness of the fish. For a very long list of topping options for baked fish check the Nutrition Chapter in my book "The Power to Heal."*

– **Fish with Lemon Caper Sauce:**

> *Sprinkle 4 fish fillets of choice with natural sea salt and sauté 4 minutes skin side up in a heated skillet coated with 1 tablespoon olive oil. Turn and cook 4 minutes or more until done. Remove from pan and keep warm in the oven. Add 2 teaspoons chopped wild organic capers to pan and sauté for 15 seconds. Left over capers can add flavor to many recipes or salads and is too often forgotten as a way of adding a taste treat to a recipe. Add ½ cup bottled clam juice for best flavor or chicken broth if allergic to shell fish. Add 1 tablespoon fresh or bottled lemon juice and boil down for about 3 minutes. Left over clam juice can be frozen for any fish or seafood future recipe. Add 2 tablespoons Better Butter, and 1 tablespoon fresh or 1 teaspoon dried parsley and pour over fish. Long green beans or asparagus makes this dish look dramatic. Serve with your favorite salad.*

– **Garlic and Pecan Crusted Fish Fillets:**

> *Preheat oven to 400 degrees. Blend 1/3 cup of pecans, very thin outer layer of one lemon (peeled with a potato peeler … or use lemon zest), 3 cloves of garlic and ½ teaspoon of sea salt in a small hand processor. Arrange about 1 pound of any mild, white fish fillet (that is bone free) on an oiled baking dish.*

Press the mixture over one side of the fish and bake about 20 minutes until fish is cooked and nuts are toasted. Serve with a fabulous salad ... enjoy!

– **Crab cakes for that special occasion we all need recipes for:**

Combine 1 pound of fresh lump crabmeat (picked over to remove cartilage) with 1 hormone and antibiotic free whisked egg, ½ cup chopped scallions (salad green onions), 2 tablespoons Spectrum Canola mayonnaise, 1 tablespoon Diijon mustard, ¼ teaspoon sea salt, 2 tablespoons any tolerated breadcrumbs (make your own in a blender with a tolerated bread). Form into cakes, and low heat sauté in 2 tablespoons of organic olive oil until brown for about 5 minutes per side. If desired you can also broil the crab cakes. Make an impressive salad and one of the special cooked vegetables listed below. You can make any cooked vegetable special by topping with roasted chopped nuts like walnuts or pecans ... or toasted sesame seeds ... and serve the dinner by candlelight.

POACHED EGGS AND GREENS:

*First steam any favorite chopped greens of choice like kale or spinach in a little water seasoned with organic garlic, fresh or dried onion, parsley and sea salt until wilted. Leave in warm water until eggs are finished. A messed up poached egg is not a pretty sight. There are some basic guidelines to a successful poached egg. Fill a wide saucepan with about two inches of water and bring to a **gentle** simmer. A rolling boil will toughen and twist the egg whites. Add two teaspoons of a tolerated vinegar (consider Coconut Secret Vinegar) that helps the eggs keep their shape. Crack the freshest eggs (that will not spread as much as older eggs) into a small container and **gently** add the eggs one at a time into the water and cook for three minutes. While the eggs are cooking drain the warm cooked greens and place on individual plates. Remove the eggs with a* *slotted spoon and place on the cooked greens. Serve immediate with an already made salad of choice.*

- **There are endless uses for hard boiled eggs** ... *but not the ones with rubbery whites, chalky yolks, and green-gray film between the yolk and white. Boiling eggs correctly in the right temperature makes all the difference. Place eggs in a saucepan with an inch or two of* **cold water** *and set the pan over high heat. When the water reaches a* **full boil** *remove from heat, cover the pan and let the eggs stand for 10 minutes. This cooks them gently and keeps the whites from toughening. If you are not using them right away set them in an ice water bath to lower the temperature and minimize the pressure that cause sulfur rings to form. Now you are ready to use in any recipe you want or just in the refrigerator for that needed snack.*

- **Ideas with white chicken meat:**

White chicken meat is lower in fat than the dark meat. You can buy chicken breasts for 3-4 meals and boil, low heat sauté or bake ... then freeze for quick easy meals like:

   * *Add chopped cooked chicken to your favorite salad combination for a cold platter.*

   * *Add chopped chicken to olive oil and stir-fry with your favorite vegetables; season with Coconut Aminos. In picking vegetables to stir-fry consider green and/or yellow summer squash, Chinese cabbage, Bok Choy, parsley, onion, garlic, celery, red or green cabbage. You can also use the more unusual vegetables like jicama or kohlrabi that are both good cooked or raw.*

   * *Add chopped chicken to your tolerated chicken broth with lots of sliced scallions, very fine cut up celery, sea salt and garlic to taste, and slowly add whipped organic eggs to make egg drop soup.*

* *Wrap cooked chicken, and desired vegetables in a romaine lettuce leaf moistened with your tolerated salad dressing.*

* *Make a hash with chopped chicken, vegetables of choice, and cooked low glycemic index quinoa. Season hash with Coconut Aminos.*

– **ROOT VEGETABLE STEW:**

Root vegetables are complex carbohydrates that break down slowly in digestion and give you a hearty meal that keeps you from getting hungry so quickly. This recipe can be varied in many ways but I'll list the basics and you make your own creation.

In one tablespoon olive oil cook 1 cup chopped onion, 3 tablespoons chopped garlic, ½ cup chopped celery with 1 tablespoon chopped fresh rosemary (or 1 teaspoon dried rosemary) and 1 teaspoon sea salt. Add 1 quart of your favorite chicken broth, non-chicken broth or vegetable broth (more if needed). Add about 2 cups each of any root vegetable like diced peeled rutabagas, diced peeled turnips, diced peeled parsnips, diced baby carrots and diced peeled sweet potatoes. Simmer until tender … serve with one of your special salads. For a thicker stew higher in protein you can add ¼ cup of spouted Quinoa, sprouted lentils and/or sprouted mung beans.

– **Quick Shrimp Chowder:**

In a medium skillet over medium–high heat, add 1 tablespoon olive oil to coat pan. Then add ½ cup chopped carrots, ½ cup chopped red or yellow onion, ¼ cup chopped celery and sauté until tender. Stir in 2 tablespoons Quinoa flour, 2 cups organic vegetable broth, 2 teaspoons minced fresh thyme (or ½ teaspoon dried) and 1 pound of medium peeled and deveined shrimp. Cover and simmer 5 minutes. Stir in 1/3 cup regular coconut milk (not lite) and simmer 4 minutes. Add sea salt if needed.

– **Crispy chicken strips:**

These snacks or party type food are loaded with extra flavor, fiber and protein. Dipped into your favorite dipping sauce they are a sure hit for any fun occasion; or consider hummus or a mixture of your favorite mustard or tahini dressing.

Cut 1 pound boneless, skinless chicken breasts into ¼ inch thick strips. Combine with 1 cup Old Chatham sheep yogurt, cover and refrigerate for 1 hour; drain and discard yogurt. Combine ½ cup breadcrumbs made from your tolerated bread in a blender, ¼ cup garbanzo bean flour (if you do not tolerate legumes substitute quinoa flour), ¼ cup chopped pecans, 2 tablespoons organic sprouted flaxseed, 1 teaspoon paprika, ½ teaspoon sea salt in a shallow pan. Dredge each yogurt soaked chicken strip in the mixture pressing firmly to coat. Heat 4 tablespoons olive oil in a large skillet over medium heat. Sauté (this is not a high heat fried food) for about 6 minute per side until golden brown. This is a great party finger food recipe that can also be baked in the oven at 350 degrees until brown.

– **Lemon Salmon with Broccoli:**

Slice ½ lemon into thin slices and set aside. Juice remaining ½ lemon into a measuring cup and add water to equal ½ cup. Add 1 tablespoon Coconut Crystals and set aside. In a skillet heat ½ tablespoon butter over medium heat. Sprinkle 4 skinless salmon fillets with sea salt and cook about 3 minutes or until bottoms are golden. Turn fillets and add lemon juice mixture. Add 1 tablespoon snipped fresh dill (or ½ teaspoon dried) and lemon slices. Cover and cook about 5 minutes until fish flakes easily. In another skillet heat 1 tablespoon olive oil. Quarter broccoli lengthwise into long spears and add to skillet with 4 fresh garlic cloves peeled and thinly sliced. Cook over medium heat about 8 minutes or until crisp-tender. Serve salmon with broccoli on the side; pour pan juices over salmon. If you have fresh dill, top salmon with more dill and serve. This makes a beautiful company or special occasion meal.

– **Best dinner for weight loss:**

The best choices for dinner eliminate the starchy foods like potatoes, sweet potatoes and all grains. Dinner should be a protein choice fixed with low glycemic index ingredients, a cooked vegetable and a raw salad.

Avoid any sugar or fruit with the evening meal. If you do not know what foods are low in glycemic index log onto glycemicindex.com. Rather than scanning lists of commercial food you do not want to purchase, you can type in the foods you want to eat and retrieve the glycemic index information. Food choices for weight loss are best picked from those foods with a glycemic index below 55.

One of your fabulous soup recipes from the freezer makes a great dinner with a salad. I cannot emphasize enough the value of making a triple amount of a special soup recipe and freezing for future meals. I find Sunday is a good soup making day if I'm home all day and I always make triple for the effort. Usually my effort feeds us for Sunday dinner and makes about four meals for the freezer. That is called multi-tasking! Always label your container with the name and date like "turkey and root veggies and the date" or "buffalo and bean and the date", or "lamb and turnips and the date."

DINNER VEGETABLES

- Bake **butternut squash** for one hour and top with Better Butter and sea salt. You can also bake or boil parsnips that are forgotten by the average cook but can be a substitute for potatoes as a side dish or in recipes. You can whip up any cooked vegetable like summer squash, zucchini, cauliflower, parsnips, broccoli with Better Butter and sea salt. Then for desired thinness, you can add non-dairy milk or lite coconut milk. If you cannot eat potatoes, whipped vegetables make a great substitute.

- Any vegetables such as **broccoli, spinach or kale** can be made special by the following:

    After steaming to desired tenderness and drained, mix with 2 teaspoons of toasted sesame oil, 2 teaspoons Coconut Aminos, 1 large minced garlic clove.

- There are many **grilled vegetable** recipes with complicated dressings in magazines, but any vegetable of choice can be grilled with your **favorite salad dressing** either in the oven or the George Foreman grill.

- Any recipe will taste better if you toast the garlic or nuts. This **Green Bean and Toasted Garlic** recipe would not taste the same with just fresh garlic added.

    Cook 1 pound of whole green beans in boiling water for 5 minutes. Plunge into cold water and drain. Add 2 teaspoons of butter, 1 teaspoon of olive oil and 4 very large garlic cloves thinly sliced and sauté for 1 minute, remove and set aside. Add cooked beans, ¼ teaspoon sea salt and cook 2 minutes. Serve topped with the toasted garlic. You can add fresh ground pepper before serving if you desire.

- **Grilled asparagus** makes a great companion to any meal but dressed up like this makes it special: Fresh asparagus season is short and the long spears are great so before you settle for short asparagus cuts, look for the frozen brand that keeps the spears long.

   Grill 1 to 1 ½ pound of asparagus coated with 1 tablespoon extra virgin olive oil and 1/4 teaspoon natural sea salt (optional) for about 4 minutes until crisp tender. Combine 1 tablespoon extra virgin olive oil, ¼ teaspoon natural sea salt with 1 tablespoon Coconut vinegar, ½ teaspoon of your favorite mustard, and 1 minced garlic clove until well blended. Stir in 2 teaspoons coarsely chopped capers (optional) and drizzle over asparagus on a serving platter. Sprinkle with ¼ cup fresh basil leaves (or 1 tablespoons organic dried basil).

   The above fancy recipe can be shorted to just broiling the asparagus spears with olive oil and sea salt. You can also use green zucchini cut into ½ inch slices.

- Some people do better if they make their own **salad dressings** because commercial dressings all seem to have at least one ingredient you do not want. Here are simple dressings you can make at home:

   *   *Take 1 cup of any nut choice and blend to a paste with ¼ cup of water. You can shorten this by using nut butter of choice. Add a tolerated oil of choice to the consistency you want. Olive oil is the best healthy oil but if you do not like a strong flavor use any tolerated oil except soy. Sesame oil is the best oil for the pancreas and digestion. Add Spectrum brand of*

Canola mayonnaise to taste. If you cannot find a commercial mayonnaise with tolerated ingredients you can Google Ener-G Egg Free mayonnaise for a recipe. Add more oil for the right consistency you want for salad dressing. If you want it tart add Coconut Vinegar. If it becomes too tart add Coconut Crystals. Vary the recipe with crushed garlic or herb of choice like tarragon or oregano. You can vary any salad dressing with lemon or lime juice, plain or roasted garlic Hummus.

* *You can make a simple salad dressing with olive oil, Coconut Vinegar and Coconut Crystals.*

* *Mix your tolerated oil like olive or sesame with Coconut Secret Coconut Aminos for a delicious salad dressing.*

* **Mix your favorite organic mustard with desired amount of tolerated vinegar (try Coconut Vinegar) and Coconut Crystals.** *Try this over finely chopped steamed kale leaves with the stems removed for a delicious vegetable many people forget to eat.*

– **Baked Spaghetti Squash:**

Cut squash in half and clean out seeds. Bake in 350 degree oven for 30–45 minutes depending on the size of the squash. Then scoop out the fleshy strands with a fork that will come out like spaghetti. Top with any favorite sauce, Better Butter, or topping of choice.

This recipe makes spaghetti squash special: Cook squash like above. Roast ¼ cup pine nuts in the oven spread out on a baking sheet while you are baking the squash for about 7–10 minutes. Check them occasionally as they can burn easily due to their high fat content. If you cannot afford pine nuts roast walnuts or pecans. In a small skillet heat 1 ½ tablespoons olive oil over medium heat and add 4 large minced garlic cloves; stir for 2 minutes. While squash is hot spoon out the strands and mix with the garlic mixture. Sprinkle the top with the roasted nuts.

- **Squash recipes:**

In a container with a lid thoroughly shake 1 cup Coconut Vinegar, ¾ cup organic olive oil, 2 tablespoons of Coconut Crystals, 1 teaspoon dried basil, 2 cloves of minced garlic and 1 teaspoon natural sea salt. Cook 4 cups of sliced zucchini about 3 minutes until tender but still crisp and drain. Place in a closed container, cover completely with dressing and chill overnight. To serve, drain zucchini and place on lettuce leaves, top with thin slices of white or red onion, and drizzle with some of the marinade.

Another marinade for summer yellow squash and green zucchini is 1 teaspoon natural sea salt, 2 tablespoons Coconut Aminos, 2 tablespoons Coconut Vinegar, 2 tablespoons of Coconut Crystals and 1 tablespoon sesame oil.

Summer yellow squash and green zucchini can be eaten raw or stir-fried. In a skillet sauté 2 pounds of sliced squash with 4 tablespoons of Better Butter, 1 large white or red onion (yellow onion is too strong for the delicate squash), 1 clove of minced garlic or organic garlic powder and natural sea salt. If you do not have a problem with the Nightshade foods you can add 1 small chopped green pepper and stir in 4 small chopped tomatoes last. Stir-fry until vegetables are almost done and serve with ¼ cup of shredded Manchego sheep cheese over the top. You can also sprinkle top with gluten free croutons.

A simple quick stir-fry with 3-4 small summer yellow squash or green zucchini is just to sauté in 2 tablespoons Better Butter, 1 tablespoon Coconut Aminos and 1-2 chopped green onions for several minutes.

Another simple quick stir-fry with 1 ½ pounds of sliced summer yellow squash and green zucchini uses 3 tablespoons olive oil, 2 chopped garlic, 1 tablespoon Coconut Vinegar, ¼ cup fresh or 1 tablespoon dried basil (or fresh or dried parsley), and natural sea salt.

Combine ½ cup any mild tasting organic oil (like canola), ½ cup Coconut Vinegar, 2 tablespoons of Coconut Crystals, ¼ teaspoon natural sea salt, 1 small sliced yellow summer squash and 1 small green zucchini, 1 small white or red onion sliced in rings. Refrigerate in a covered container for several hours.

A small striped yellow and green oblong squash is called **Delicata squash**. *It can be cut open and seeds removed and then sliced very thin (including the skin). Coat the slices with a little olive oil and sea salt and place the slices in a single layer on an oiled cookie sheet. One option is to sprinkle with a very thin layer of cinnamon with or without Coconut Crystals. You can also roast it with thin slices of red onion and rosemary. Bake at 350 degrees until tender – about 30 minutes. This unusual squash is always a hit and so easy to make because you eat the thin skin and all. You can also cook it in stir-fries or steamed and tossed with roasted nuts. Once you realize how easy it to cook you can change the seasoning in dozens of ways.*

DESSERTS

The best dessert recipe is to take one of your favorites and try to adjust the ingredients to be lower in sugar and carbohydrates.

Substitute Quinoa or Teff for wheat.

Substitute Coconut Crystals for sugar.

Substitute Coconut Nectar for maple syrup, honey or agave.

Substitute Old Chatam sheep yogurt for cow yogurt.

Substitute regular coconut milk for heavy cream.

Substitute lite coconut milk, dairy-free almond milk, rice milk or hemp milk for dairy.

Substitute Coconut ice cream for dairy ice cream (some brands are soy free).

Use organic ingredients.

Make bread crumbs in your blender with tolerated bread.

Consider the **cookie** recipe on the back of the Teff flour package and *use any combination of quinoa, coconut, millet and teff flours. Use Coconut Nectar for maple syrup.*

Fudge is easy to make using ½ of a *100% unsweetened chocolate baking bar and sweeten with 1 cup Coconut Crystals, 1 can of regular coconut milk (not lite), 2 teaspoons organic Vanilla and ½ cup of chopped* *nuts. If you want it sweeter you can add a few scoops of Stevia. Heat all ingredients together (but not to boil) and spread in an oiled glass baking pan and chill. Cut into squares. If product is too thin and does not sit up for fudge consistency it is delicious spread over Coconut ice cream or make* **cupcakes** *out of the muffin recipe on the Teff package. Substitute Quinoa flour for rice flour and Coconut Nectar for brown sugar. Then spread fudge recipe over top for icing.*

Coconut Flour Fudge Brownies are easy to make and the coconut flour adds a blast of fiber to these chewy brownies. If you want them extra gooey just bake less time.

> *Preheat oven to 325 degrees, butter and flour an 8 inch square baking dish. Melt 1 stick organic butter and 6 ounces 100% baking chocolate over low heat until smooth. Whisk in ½ cup Coconut Crystals, ½ cup Coconut Nectar, 1 tablespoon organic vanilla, 3 large hormone and antibiotic free eggs, and 1 tablespoon water. Stir in ½ cup loosely packed coconut flour and ¼ teaspoon sea salt. Pour batter into baking dish and bake 30 minutes or until a toothpick comes out clean. Cook before cutting into squares and store in the refrigerator.*

Quinoa makes a great pudding. *1 cup of well rinsed white, black or red quinoa (or a mixture) added to 2 cups of boiling water and ½ teaspoon sea salt, then simmer for 15 minutes or until soft. Drain off any excess water and add 1 cup of non-dairy unsweetened milk (or more if you want it soupier), 1 tablespoon butter, 3 tablespoons Coconut Nectar, ½ teaspoon cinnamon. Serve in a shallow bowl dusted with additional cinnamon and ¼ cup of toasted almonds or chopped pecans.*

Tapioca makes a great pudding. *In a saucepan simmer 2 cups of dairy free unsweetened milk or lite coconut milk, 1/3 cup organic quick cooking granulated Tapioca, ¼ teaspoon sea salt, 2 tablespoons Coconut Crystals for about 15 minutes while stirring often. You can top with organic shredded coconut or organic seasonal fruit ... or blueberry compote.*

And, understand that occasionally you just need to treat yourself like a birthday or an anniversary. For special occasions take a small serving just to taste instead of a normal serving. I know a lady on a weight loss program who ordered a piece of chocolate cake and did not eat it but smelled it for one hour. That stress only messed up her adrenal glands. She would have been better off to have taken a very small slice and enjoyed a few bites. **When it comes to desserts pass unless it is really important, and substitute when you can.** *A weight loss program does not have to be like having a tooth pulled without anesthesia.* **Be proud of the changes you make, and be reasonable in all other situations.**

ENJOY YOUR JOURNEY! REMIND YOURSELF EVERYDAY THAT YOU ARE BEAUTIFUL INSIDE AND OUT. BE RESPECTFUL OF WHAT YOU PUT INTO YOUR BODY AND THE MAGIC OF HEALTH ... NOT JUST WEIGHT LOSS ... WILL BE YOUR REWARD!

FINAL NOTE

This is the end of a wonderful journey together. You have learned a lot more than how to achieve weight loss. You have learned how to assume responsibility for your wellness and also the wellness of your loved ones. The best advice I can give you at this point is to have a circle of friends that support your wellness effort. They do not have to be overweight but they do have to support your belief system that overweight is a result of poor choices … and is a symptom of how you treat your body. *You can even improve your hereditary weakness by the **choices** you make in **your** lifetime.* This quote encourages you to have a support circle of family and/or friends around you that understands your energized and healthy journey, and might add information that could make that journey easier.

"I not only use all the brains that I have, but all that I can borrow."

-Woodrow Wilson, 28th President of the U.S.

ENJOY YOUR POTENTIAL!!!

ENJOY YOUR JOURNEY!!!

Made in the USA
Columbia, SC
27 January 2020